AF323615

Vol. 3
Series on Biomaterials and Bioengineering

Service Characteristics of Biomedical Materials and Implants

SERIES ON BIOMATERIALS AND BIOENGINEERING

Series Editors: **A W Batchelor** (Monash Univ. Sunway Campus Malaysia Sdn Bhd)
J R Batchelor (UK)
Margam Chandrasekaran (Singapore Institute of Manufacturing Technology, Singapore)

Series on Biomaterials and Bioengineering — Vol. 3

Service Characteristics of Biomedical Materials and Implants

Andrew W Batchelor
Monash University, Malaysia

Margam Chandrasekaran
Singapore Institute of Manufacturing Technology, Singapore

Imperial College Press

Published by

Imperial College Press
57 Shelton Street
Covent Garden
London WC2H 9HE

Distributed by

World Scientific Publishing Co. Pte. Ltd.
5 Toh Tuck Link, Singapore 596224
USA office: Suite 202, 1060 Main Street, River Edge, NJ 07661
UK office: 57 Shelton Street, Covent Garden, London WC2H 9HE

British Library Cataloguing-in-Publication Data
A catalogue record for this book is available from the British Library.

SERVICE CHARACTERISTICS OF BIOMEDICAL MATERIALS AND IMPLANTS
Series on Biomaterials and Bioengineering — Vol. 3

Copyright © 2004 by Imperial College Press

ISBN   1-86094-475-2

Printed by FuIsland Offset Printing (S) Pte Ltd, Singapore

Dedicated to

Mrs. Valli Boobal Batchelor

Shri Comal Neelakantan Margam and Shrimathi Rajeswari Margam

Preface

This book grew out of the realization during experimental research about how little is known concerning the service conditions for many implants. Basic information such as the temperature rise on the surface of an orthopaedic implant during vigorous exercise is not known to any great accuracy. However, many fascinating and valuable experimental and theoretical investigations have provided at least a partial picture of processes occurring around an implanted biomaterial.

With the increasing range of prostheses and implants available to patients and the rapidly growing level of interest in tissue engineering, it became evident that an introductory text on the service characteristics of biomaterials would be helpful to students and general readers. Information that is distributed around many journals and conferences could be collated and summarized for the benefit of new students to the subject. Due to space limitations, the cited references provide only a selection of the newer publications, if any worker in this field feels neglected, the authors offer their apologies.

This is an interdisciplinary subject involving specialists in materials, medical science as well as engineering. It is not often appreciated how different the operating conditions are inside the body from what is typically expected of engineering components. An early example is the synovial joint; because healthy synovial joints enjoy low friction, it was expected that artificial synovial implants would also achieve low friction.

Some workers expressed surprise when synovial fluid failed to lubricate artificial materials effectively. Later investigations revealed the significance of the proteins in synovial fluid, where a hitherto unrecognized mechanism of lubrication prevailed.

This book aims to provide a general introduction into the main characteristics of any biomaterial after its implantation in the human body. A careful study of the contents of this book will help the reader to attempt to answer such vital questions as: Will the biomaterial disintegrate prematurely? Will the biomaterial initiate a toxic or inflammatory response in the body? How long can the service life of an implant material be extended?

The basic concepts of Materials Degradation, i.e. corrosion, wear, oxidative corrosion and other mechanisms are described in *Materials Degradation and its Control by Surface Engineering (Imperial College Press)*, this book assumes some knowledge of the basic concepts in Materials Degradation. However, as is explained in this book, the body imposes its own unique requirements of materials that would not normally be encountered elsewhere. The long-term service requirements of biomaterials are also much more demanding than is the case for machinery.

The book is intended for final year undergraduates, post-graduates who are pursuing a course in biomaterials or biomedical engineering. Professional engineers or scientists involved in such problems as e.g., the design of hip prostheses, may also find the book useful.

Acknowledgements

The authors would like to acknowledge the support of Monash University Malaysia and the Singapore Institute of Manufacturing Technology, Singapore. The authors would also like to record their appreciation of the following persons for their kind provision of drawings and photographs in this book: Dr. Rajaraman, Surgical Oncologist, Chennai, India, for the photographs of the elbow prosthesis, before and during its surgical implantation, Dr Tom Joyce of the University of Durham (Great Britain) for photographs of the finger prosthesis and its test apparatus (Figures A2.1, A2.2 and A2.3, Appendix 2, Dr Stephen Hsu of the National Institute of Standards and Technology, United States of America for colour drawings of arthritic synovial joints (Figure 1.1) and orthopaedic implants for the hip(Figure 1.2), for the knee prosthesis (cover page) and for photographs of hip and knee implants (Figures 4.4), Dr Wolfgang Kerkhoffs of the Helmholtz-Institute for Biomedical Engineering, University of Technology Aachen, Germany for soliciting Figures A2.4, A2.5 and for providing Figure A2.6. Figures A2.4 and A2.5 were kindly provided by Prof. Dipl.Ing. Dr. Kurt P. Judmann and Dipl.-Ing. Georg Reinisch of Vienna University of Technology and the BMF Biomechanische Forschungs-Gesellschaft m.b.H Rechte Wienzeile 5/2 A 1040 Vienna, Austria.

The efforts of Dr. Tom Joyce (Chapter 4), Dr Neo Tee Khin, external lecturer of National University of Singapore, (Chapter 6) to review the book are also acknowledged with appreciation by the authors. The reviews of Chapters 1, 2 and 3 by Prof. J.R. Batchelor, Imperial College of Science, Technology and Medicine are gratefully appreciated. Reviews of Dr. Anders Eric Jarffors, Senior Scientist, Singapore Institute of Manufacturing Technology for Chapters 7-9 and Dr. Anil Kishen, Asst. Professor, NUS for chapters 10-12 are also acknowledged with thanks. In Chapter 5, the reviews by Dr Wolfgang Kerkhoffs, Dr Takehisa Matsuda (Department of Biomedical Engineering, Graduate School of Medical Sciences, Kyushu University, Japan) and Dr Naren Vyavahare, Associate Professor of Bioengineering, Clemson University, South Carolina, USA are acknowledged with appreciation. In Chapter 3, the helpful comments of Prof. Nicholas Spencer, The Swiss Federal Institute of Technology, are also acknowledged.

The authors also wish to acknowledge the help rendered by Mrs. Valli Boobal Batchelor and Mrs. Lakshmi Chandrasekaran for editing the manuscript. The authors also acknowledge with thanks the encouragement and support of their family members during the writing of this book.

Contents

Chapter 1

Introduction

1.1 Definitions and requirements of biomedical implants

A biomedical implant is defined in simple terms as an artificial organ used for restoring the functionality of a damaged natural organ or tissue of the body. In other words it is expected to perform the functions of the natural organ or tissue without adverse effect to other parts of the body. This calls for various requirements to be satisfied by the artificial organ or the material used for the artificial organ construction before it can be considered for application. The basic requirement of the artificial organ or tissue substitute is that it should act as a functional replacement for the original body part. The additional requirements include Biocompatibility or the Biodegradability of the material used in the artificial organ so that the surrounding tissue accommodates it without any immune rejection response or inflammatory reaction. Another application of materials in the biomedical engineering field are the drug delivery systems where the required drug is enclosed in a capsule, which is fed to the patient and the drug is later released to the desired location in the body.

1.1.1 *Biocompatibility and biodegradability*

Biocompatibility and Biodegradability are the two concepts that are closely associated with the biomedical engineering. 'Biocompatibility' is to indicate the immune rejection responses of the surrounding tissue systems to the presence of a foreign object in the body. The basic

1

requirement of any artificial implant is that it should not to generate immune-rejection or inflammatory responses. Another class of materials frequently used in biomedical implants is the biodegradable or bio-absorbable materials in applications requiring temporary presence in the body. A typical example of an implant could be bone fracture fixation devices. After the healing process is completed the fixation devices could cause discomfort to the patient and warrant removal of the device. For similar reasons, any drug delivery system needs to be biodegradable. The drugs are sealed in a capsule usually made of a polymer and upon release of the drug at the desired location, the capsule is expected to degrade so that it does not trigger a foreign object immune rejection response in the surrounding tissue membranes. There are certain physical property requirements for such biodegradable/ bio-absorbable implants such as high initial strength, high initial modulus and controlled strength and modulus retention *in vivo* so that it could provide the necessary support or augment the capacity of the tissue to regenerate. Research is focused on developing a true biocompatible material, which can undergo biodegradation or promote faster healing, by tissue in-growth. The service characteristics of a material, e.g. its rate of degradation in the tissues or the rate of wear, have a strong influence on the biocompatibility of an implant made of the same material.

1.2 History of development of biomedical materials and implants

The development of biomedical materials closely coincided with the beginnings of surgery. The ancient Egyptians are known to have used prostheses to substitute for amputated limbs. At approximately 1000 BC, a mature lady who may have lost her big toe through gangrene was fitted with wooden prostheses to replace the big toe [Nerhlich et al.]. The prosthesis was skillfully sculpted to closely resemble a big toe and was able to flex relative to the foot.   This is the earliest known surviving example of a prosthesis fitted to a recipient, who was alive at the time of the surgical placement (although only the mummified remains of the lady exist today).   It was also the practice of those times to fit prostheses to bodies intended for mummification [Nerhlich et al.]. Wood would have been suitable for use in prosthesis, because of its high strength to weight ratio and toughness.   There is also mention in the Veda period of ancient Indian literature (1500 to 1800 BC) that artificial legs, eyes and teeth were used at that time [Goh].

With the invention of anaesthesia, it became possible to fit implants inside the human body. Metal plates could be attached by screws to the fractured ends of bones, thus repairing complex fractures. Problems of stiff joints and arthritis received attention in the mid-20th century when Philip Wiles, working in London, United Kingdom, developed an articulating metal joint that could be implanted inside a hip [Amstutz and Grigoris]. This all-metal implant was later followed in 1962 by the design of Sir John Charnley, which combined polymer and metal components. These hip prostheses were intended to closely simulate the original hip joint and consisted of a separate 'cup' and a ball joined to a stem for securing this part of the prosthesis inside the femur bone. The implanted joint retained almost the same freedom of movement as the original joint. The Charnley prosthesis was particularly successful, providing mobility for thousands of patients. The success of the Charnley implant and other designs lead to the release of many competing designs of 'artificial joint', which offered greater freedom of movement, were easier for surgeons to implant or presented less post-operative difficulties [Amstutz and Grigoris].

Not all implants were developed to improve the health of a patient, the human need to appear youthful and attractive have provided the motivation to develop several distinctive types of implant. The mid to late 20th century was the period when women especially began to use biomedical materials for aesthetic reasons. Cosmetic surgery of the breasts often involves the implantation of a soft polymer capsule filled with silicone oil. This implant presented a major challenge to the development engineers since there was a risk of leakage of silicone oil into the body. For the male patients, penile implants are popular where an elastic polymer is used to provide resilient support to combat impotence.

As expectations of health increased in parallel with rising affluence, researchers began to study how other types of implants might help ameliorate a wider range of health problems. Common medical problems such as arthritis and cardiac infarct have become amenable to treatment by implants. By inserting a tube down the artery, the blocked arteries of a cardiac infarct can be opened. In locations outside of the heart, a tube may be used to establish a 'bypass' of the blood vessel. The tube is often made of non-degradable plastic. The ageing of most populations in advanced societies has lead to a very rapid increase in the demand for biomedical implants by patients seeking to maintain a vigorous lifestyle until the end of their lives. Most governments or public health bodies of advanced countries are also very interested in implants, which help people to remain independent and productive for a greater part of their lives. The combined demands of a longer human life span and a longer fraction of the life span with an active lifestyle, have lead to a need for high performance biomedical materials that can last for up to e.g., 30 years for orthopaedic implants [Chevalier, *see* Adam]. One of the most common complaints that reduces the mobility and dexterity of patients is arthritis, either as rheumatoid arthritis or osteo-arthritis, this is illustrated schematically in Figure 1.1

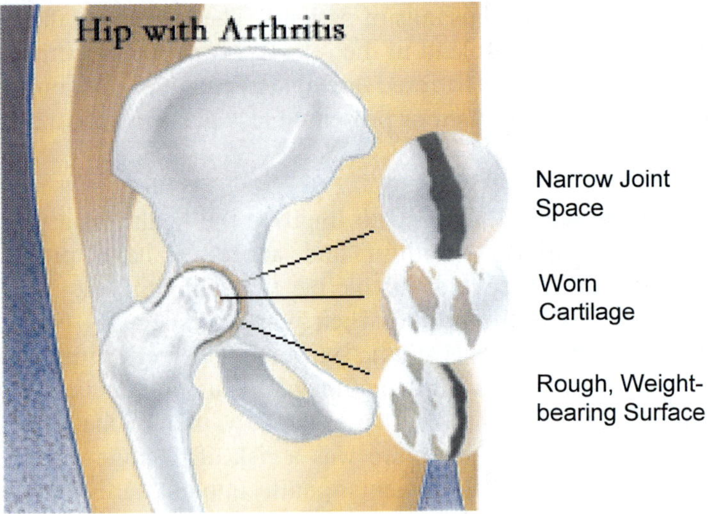

Fig 1.1. The mechanism of arthritis: a very wide spread problem that implants are used to control. Picture by courtesy of Dr Stephen Hsu, National Institute of Standards and Technology, United States of America.

1.3   The range of biomedical materials and implants

Metals, ceramics, polymers and natural materials have all been used for biomedical implants. The need to avoid toxic materials has caused aluminium or its alloys to be rarely used while plain steel would corrode too rapidly to be used in the body. High quality metal alloys of titanium, vanadium and chromium are commonly used for orthopaedic prostheses (artificial joints) or for fixing plates to correct fractures. Engineering ceramics such as aluminium oxide have been found to provide a hard, low friction surface that is also suitable for orthopaedic prostheses. In many cases, the hard aluminium oxide is paired with the much softer, but wear-resistant polymer, Ultra-High Molecular-Weight Polyethylene to produce a very durable cup and ball joint for hip joint prosthesis. Natural materials such as pig's cartilage are used for artificial heart valves after chemical denaturing to prevent allergic response by the human body.

Composite materials have attracted interest as biomedical materials. Carbon-fibre weaves have studied as reinforcing materials for the stems of orthopaedic implants. Surface coatings have been developed as a means of sheathing a metal in a coating that is more acceptable to the human body. Metals in elemental form are essentially alien to the human body. When a metal implant is inserted in tissue, most metals become encapsulated by a thin layer, which is almost empty of human cells. Adhesion between the metal implant and the surrounding tissue is comparatively weak. Bones contain 'calcium hydroxyapatite' (a form of calcium phosphate) as a structural matrix. When a metal implant is coated with hydroxyapatite, bone cells adhere onto the surface of the apatite coating without any intervening layer. The 'calcium hydroxyapatite' matrix of the bone cells later becomes integral with the hydroxyapatite coating and there is excellent adhesion of the coated implant to the bone.

The range of biomedical materials is expanding very rapidly; there is a rapidly widening range of polymer materials proposed as biomaterials. Biocomposites, i.e. composite materials intended for use as biomaterials also add to the range of potential materials. Composite materials are now developing beyond the relatively simple structure of two perhaps to three materials to systems which have an engineered structure at the nanometre scale. Vacuum-based surface coating technologies such as Physical Vapour Deposition are used to create regular arrays of polysaccharide molecules on a supporting membrane of polymer. The purpose of this composite biomedical material is to selectively adsorb specific proteins and reject other proteins. This material can be coupled to electrodes to form a sensor for individual proteins [Shi et al.].

Due to the enormous range of biomaterials, materials are not described individually in this book, instead the various types of implants are discussed and critical service characteristics of materials are illustrated. Materials typically used to fulfill such service characteristics, e.g. titanium alloys for orthopaedic implants, are mentioned at this point.

The fundamental function of a biomedical material is also changing. The original form of biomedical implant was a discrete quantity of material such as a plate to link fractured bones. While this type of implant is likely to remain in use for the conceivable future, a new form of implant is rapidly gaining prominence. High porosity implants, often referred to as 'scaffolds', serve as matrices to foster cell growth or re-growth where the original tissue is defective. Vital material properties for these 'scaffolds' are flexibility and permeability so that the cells within are not shielded from the mechanical stresses imposed on tissues nor is excluded from the natural flow of cellular nutrients. Mechanical stress is found to be necessary for cell growth in tissues such as arterial and vein walls. If the scaffold is made of a natural material, it may even serve as a nutrient for the cells. Effectively designed scaffolds can enable tissue regeneration in orthopaedic joints, intestines and arterial walls [Senior]. Regenerated tissue is often far more acceptable to the patient than having to live with an implant of artificial material that is entirely different from tissue.

While in most cases, the biomedical material is intended to last at least as long as the probable remaining life of the patient, some biomedical materials are designed to degrade quickly. Rapid degradation is useful where it is intended that the implant provide mechanical support to injured tissue until tissue repair is complete. A recent example of this is the polylactate polymer, which can be woven into fibres to provide a matrix for cartilage tissue recovery. This matrix is an example of the 'scaffold' discussed above. After the cartilage is recovered, enzymes in the human body decompose the polylactate. Another application of accelerated materials degradation is drug delivery. An antibiotic or pharmaceutical medicine can be coated with a degradable organic polymer, which contains a standard amount of the drug prevents contamination. Some drugs can be destroyed by gastric acid inside the stomach, so the coating is made resistant to acidic but not alkaline conditions. This allows the pill to survive passage through the stomach before the coating dissolves in the alkaline milieu of the small intestine to release the drug.

Another class of biomedical materials may only have a very short residence time in the body before they are removed. Stitches and sutures belong to this category of biomedical implants, but perhaps the shortest residence time is found in latex moulding material. When an orthopaedic surgeon hollows out the end of a hipbone before inserting an implant, a plastic bag filled with latex is squeezed into the hole. By pressurizing the latex an accurate casting of the hole can be obtained. The flexibility of latex allows it to be pulled out after solidification. The latex casting is then measured to allow the immediate manufacture of an optimally sized stem to the hip implant [Mulier]. Progressive loosening of improperly sized implants is reported to be effectively prevented by this technique.

Highly topical developments in miniature cameras such as those, which can roam within a patient's gastro-intestinal tract, [Taylor; Scapa et al.] pose new demands on biomedical materials. The camera should be enclosed by materials, which can survive the acidity of the stomach, and avoid irritation of the stomach walls or internal surfaces of the intestines and colon. In most cases the camera is designed to spend only a few hours in the digestive system, but contingency should be allowed for the occasion where the camera becomes trapped inside the digestive system. Some materials may be initially benign but subsequently damage or irritate tissues after prolonged contact.

Biomedical materials do not always have to be used as implants; instead a biomedical device could function in close contact with the exterior of the body. An important example of this is contact lenses, where a flexible glass disc resides on the exterior of the cornea. The interface between the glass disc and the lens provides a niche for bacterial or viral infection. Inflammation of the eye by the use of contact lens is still a major health problem since the duration of continuous usage without cleaning is increasing [Dart].

1.3.1 *Biomedical implants as active mediators of tissue growth*

Until recently, biomedical materials have been considered to have primarily a structural function or an optical function for opthalmic implants. Interaction between the human cells and the biomedical material has been viewed as a matter of accommodation rather than inter-related function. A clear example of this limited interaction is the hydroxyapatite-coated metal implant where the metal core is unaffected by the incorporation of the hydroxyapatite coating into the surrounding bone. Human cells are almost certainly more efficient than artificial materials for any physiological function. While solid metals may be suitable for rigid applications such as bone support, entirely different materials would be required for dynamic applications such as an artificial heart. The growing need for replacement human organs and the chronic scarcity of suitable transplants has lead researchers to seriously consider a tissue culture system that could generate replacement organs. To try and satisfy this need, the degradable 'scaffolds' described above are being transformed in scope, composition and function [McCarthy]. In its original form, the scaffold merely provides temporary structural support for human cells until they can form useful tissue. It is now realized that the scaffold is a primitive form of extra-cellular matrix. Extra-cellular matrices are known to control cell growth and cell orientation as well as provide structural support. A fully formed tissue will have required at some stage in its development the presence of an extra-cellular matrix [McCarthy]. For instance, a regular array of the extra-cellular protein laminin is required for myocytes (muscle cells) to be cultured to form a sheet of muscle. The extra-cellular matrix is known to provide nutrition and signals for specific modes of cellular development. If this extra-cellular matrix can be recreated artificially then it may be possible to grow functional tissues. These tissues would be then be implanted by the surgeon into the patient. In future therefore, the overall concept of biomedical materials may change fundamentally from the present image of self-contained inanimate materials. There are also studies into the enhancement of permanent implants, such as stents (a hollow tube designed to open a blocked artery), by depositing genetic material on the surface of the implant [Morris]. This brings gene therapy in a highly localized form to the artery where it may be possible to prevent restenosis (renewed blockage) of the artery. The relationship between the traditional functions of a biomedical implant and the newly envisaged functions are shown schematically in Figure 1.2.

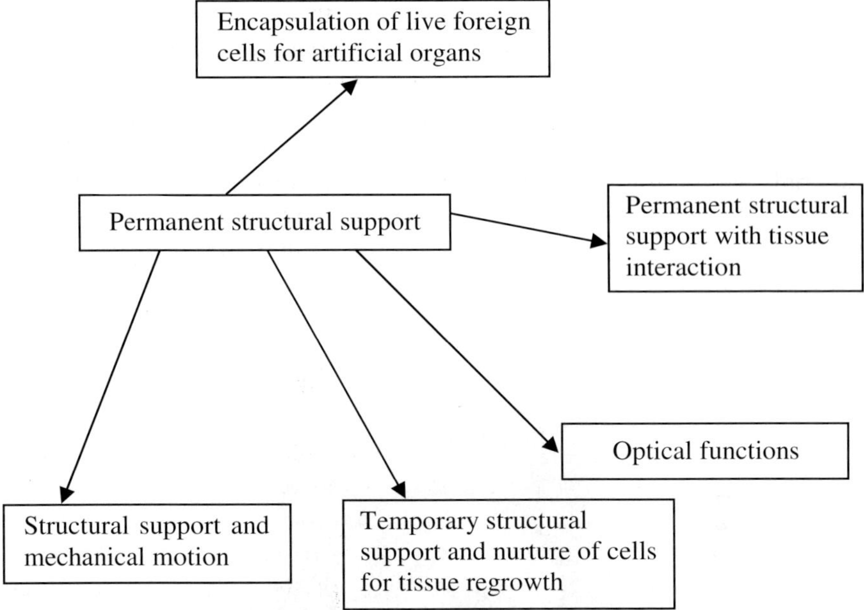

Fig 1.2. Relationship between the various functions of biomedical implants.

Surgical tools and the increasingly popular 'patches', which deliver drugs by absorption through the skin, depend on materials, which must be compatible with the human body. Although the residence time of surgical tools inside the body is comparatively short, it is still important for the tool to be non-toxic, sterile and without risk of generating allergy. The material used to form a 'patch' should not cause irritation of the human skin since the patch has to remain on the skin for a considerable period of time.

1.4 Service problems of biomedical materials

The human body poses comparatively severe conditions for most biomedical materials. The health and indeed safety of a user may depend upon the reliability of the implant. Performance limitations of biomedical materials are a perennial problem. For instance, an artificial heart-valve was implanted in more than 80,000 patients before service problems forced a recall of the heart-valve. In-service failure was caused by fatigue fracture of the struts supporting the valve flap; this contributed to the death of approximately 1,000 users [Piehler].

The implant not only has to continue to function within the human body, there should also be an absence of side effects engendered by the implant's presence. Any implant containing a sliding or impacting interface (heart-valve) will almost certainly release wear particles. Unless the implant is made of a truly inert material, some corrosion will probably occur. The body has only a limited tolerance for corrosion products and wear-particles released by an implant. A major problem with orthopaedic implants is the release of wear-particles from the moving surfaces. Perhaps the most important type of implant, certainly the implant with the highest load capacity is the hip implant, which is illustrated in Figure 1.3.

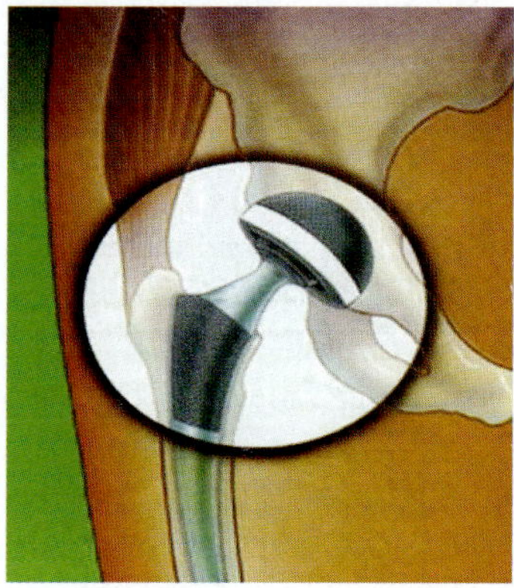

Fig 1.3. The hip implant, this implant has given some users 20 years of service without any maintenance (since this would almost certainly involve more surgery). Picture by courtesy of Dr Stephen Hsu, National Institute of Standards and Technology, USA.

Fine metal particles and oxides or hydroxides of metals such as chromium and titanium have been observed to cause inflammation, swelling and possibly even cancer in some patients. The implant should ideally last the lifetime of the user since few people would wish to regularly experience surgery for the replacement of an implant. The body generates a hostile corrosive environment to most materials that are commonly available since body fluids are largely composed of salt water. The enzymes and proteins present in tissue fluids are observed to amplify the corrosive nature of the tissue fluids. If there is inflammation around the implant, then the implant environment becomes even more corrosive because of the secretion of strong oxidants by the human cells that initiate the inflammation. There are also the requirements of high strength, high toughness and low density to ensure that the implant does not entail excessive extra weight. Heightened expectations by patients of maintaining high levels of physical activity are placing additional demands on the performance of orthopaedic implants in particular.

It is not sufficient for a material to be merely non-toxic; the material should not initiate an immune or inflammatory response from the human body nor function as a protected niche for bacterial infections. Control of the immune response is particularly important for the heart-lung machine and kidney dialysis where live blood is conveyed outside of the body through tubes and pumps. The polymers used in the tubing can activate the white blood cells inside the blood causing them to attack human tissues when the blood returns to the human body. Each time a biomedical material is inserted in the body, there is always a risk that bacteria will be conveyed into the body on the surface of the biomedical material. Intra-vascular devices (implants relating to the heart and to arteries) are very prone to this problem [Proctor]. Implants with a complex or closed form, such as a tube present much difficulty when ensuring complete sterilization of the implant. Sterility problems are not limited to implants, nor are the risks limited to bacterial or viral infection. The contemporary epidemic of variant Creutzfeldt-Jakob disease (vCJD) has generated new risks in surgical operations. The infective agent of vCJD, prions, are extremely difficult to destroy by conventional sterilization, this means that prions could be transmitted from an infected patient to other patients via contaminated surgical tools [Coghlan]. It may be necessary to develop a coating on the tool surface that is resistant to contamination by prions.

Whenever a biomedical material is inserted in the body, adsorbed proteins will almost inevitably cover this material. In some cases, this protein adsorption may lead to blood clotting, especially when fibrinogen (a protein found in blood) is involved. Fibrinogen adsorption on polymer surfaces is known to be a cause of blood clotting. Polymer linings of tubes are often coated with heparin to suppress clotting. If clotting occurs then a lump of clotted blood could block an artery causing a thrombosis.

1.5 Prediction of service life of implants

It is often difficult to predict how a biomedical material will perform over several decades of a patient's life where the physical-chemical environment may vary significantly as the patient ages. Phenomena such as wear rates after millions of sliding cycles or corrosion after a decade or more of implantation cannot be easily predicted from short-term tests. Orthopaedic implants are expected to last for approximately 15 years before excessive wear of the implant occurs [Hargreaves]. The formulation of accurate tests also requires much care, as it is not easy to reproduce in a test apparatus the conditions occurring within the human body. For example, the testing of the wear of dental implants is based on a specialized apparatus, which is designed to simulate chewing [Teoh et al.]. Detailed experimental studies have revealed how e.g., wear rates can abruptly change after a sustained period of testing. This means that extrapolation of implant life from short-term measurements would be inaccurate. There are no precise theoretical models of the service-life of an implant; some experimental data is always required to estimate the service-life. Despite the numerous tests now applied to biomedical implants, new materials continue to cause unforeseen problems in patients, often necessitating removal of the implant [Hukins, *see* Adam]. A National Institutes of Health panel has concluded that the service characteristics of implants and biomedical materials after implantation is a topic of critical importance, which remains poorly understood [Lefevre].

1.5.1 *Disposal of biomedical materials*

The volume of biomedical materials is continually increasing and is beginning to create a materials disposal problem. Implants and other biomedical materials, such as surgical gloves, are not always designed for ease of disposal after use. In the future, biomedical materials may be selected not only for service life characteristics but also for safe disposal.

1.6 Structure of this book

In chapters 2 and 3, the nature of the internal body environment and changes caused by the implantation of foreign materials is discussed. Chapters 4, 5 and 6 discuss the monolithic implants and restorative materials used in orthopaedic, cardiac and dental surgery respectively. In these chapters issues such as wear and corrosion of the implants as well as problems of tissue inflammation around the implant are discussed. The more modern types of implants, scaffolds, and containment membranes for 'artificial organs' and matrices for drug delivery systems are discussed in Chapters 7 to 10. Chapter 11 discusses materials for external medical devices, such as surgical gloves while chapter 12 looks at the problem of disposal of used biomedical materials and interactions of biomedical implants with X-rays and other modes of tissue imaging.

1.7 Summary

Biomedical materials are typically engineering materials, which have been adapted to the conditions prevailing in the human body. Development of biomedical materials began more than 100 years ago but most materials have only been developed in the past 50 years. The changing nature of human society and lifestyle expectations will ensure a growing need for a yet wider variety of biomedical materials, which perform to yet higher standards.

References

D.Adam, Techology: longer lasting hips?, *Nature Science Update*, Friday 24 November 2000.

H.C. Amstutz and P. Grigoris, Metal on Metal Bearings in Hip Arthroplasty, *Clinical Orthopaedics and Related Research*, August 1996, Vol. 329S (Supplement), pp. S11-S34.

A. Coghlan, Tonsil fear, *New Scientist*, News, 10th November 2000.

J. Dart, Extended-wear contact lenses, microbial keratitis and public health, *The Lancet*, 17 July 1999, Vol. 354, No. 9174.

James C.H. Goh, New Challenges beyond computer-aided prosthetic socket design and manufacturing, *Proc. 10th International Conference on Biomedical engineering*, 6-9 Dec. 2000, Singapore, ed.. JCH Goh, publ. National University of Singapore, pp. 61-62.

S. Hargreaves, It's hip to be smooth, *The Lancet*, 25th November 2000,'Science and Medicine'.

Greg Lefevre, Hip replacement patients may face more surgery, http://www.cnn.com/2001/HEALTH/01/17/hip.replacement

M. McCarthy, Bioengineers bring a new slant to stem-cell research, *Lancet,* 28 October 2000, Vol. 356, No. 9240, feature article.

K. Morris, Gene-coated stents herald hope for restenosis prevention, *The Lancet,* Science and medicine, 4 November 2000, Vol. 356, No. 9241.

M. Mulier, A system for intra-operative manufacturing of stems of total hip replacements, *Computer technology in Biomaterials Science and Engineering*, ed. J. Vander Sloten, publ. John Wiley and Sons, 2000.

A.G. Nerlich, A. Zink, U. Szeimies, H.J. Hagedorn, Ancient Egyptian prosthesis of the big toe, *The Lancet*, 2000, Vol. 356, pp. 2176-79.

H. R. Piehler, The Future of Medicine: Biomaterials, *Materials Research Society Bulletin*, August 2000, pp. 67-70.

R.A. Proctor, Towards an understanding of biomaterial infections: A complex interplay between the host and bacteria, Journal of Laboratory and Clinical Medicine, January 2000, Vol. 135, No. 1, pp. 14-15.

K. Senior, Artificial implants: making the marriage work, *The Lancet*, 14th August 1999, Vol. 354, No. 9178.

E. Scapa, H. Jacob, S. Lewkowicz, M. Migdal, D. Gat, A. Gluckovski, N. Gutmann and Z. Fireman, Initial experience of wireless-capsule endoscopy for evaluating occult gastrointestinal bleeding and suspected small bowel pathology, *The American Journal of Gastroenterology*, 2002, Vol. 97, No. 11, pp. 2776-2779.

H. Shi, W-B. Tsai, M.D. Garrison, S. Ferrari and B.D. Ratner, Template-imprinted nanostructured surfaces for protein recognition, *Nature*, 15 April 1999, Vol. 398, No. 6728, pp. 593-597.

C. Taylor, Pill-cam, *National Nine (Australia) Health News*, 18 October 2000.

S.H. Teoh, L.F.K.L. Ong, A.U.J. Yap and G.W. Hastings, Bruxing-type dental wear simulator for ranking of dental restorative materials, Journal of Biomedical materials Research, 1998, Vol. 43, No. 2, pp. 175-183.

Chapter 2

Physiological Environment of the Human Body

2.1 Introduction

Early life forms were believed to have evolved in the sea and adapted seawater as a body fluid. The mineral composition of human serum is surprisingly close to seawater despite the millions of years of evolution that separate early life from humans. A basic study of corrosion reveals that seawater is considered to be a corrosive liquid to most metals in common use. The human body operates at a temperature close to 37 degrees Celsius, which is a sufficiently high temperature to initiate many chemical reactions. The state of being alive depends upon a large range of chemical reactions, some happening within cells and others occurring outside of the cells. The types of biochemical reagents and enzymes, prevailing reaction paths and their mediation by the cells can be considered as the physiological environment of the human body. Any implanted biomaterial has to function within this physiological environment as it is not possible to separate an implant from the body. The characteristics of the physiological environment largely determine whether a material can be used as a biomedical material.

2.2 Physical and chemical environment

2.2.1 *The physical environment*

The physical environment is defined in terms of the temperature, pressure and stresses, radiation and vibration levels. Human beings have a limited tolerance for variations in the physical environment of pressure, temperature, vibration and radiation. A possible exception is the working environment of deep-sea divers where the water pressure on body tissues can reach 1 MPa or more. The divers however only spend a small portion of their lifetime in this pressurized environment. Most parts of the body operate in a similar physical environment with a quasi-constant temperature of approximately 37 degrees Celsius, 1 atmosphere pressure with low levels of vibration and radiation. Major exceptions to this norm include the skin, which is subject to mechanical abrasion, solar radiation and temperature and humidity variation. Mechanical stress is probably the most variable parameter of the physical environment in the human body. The skeleton, synovial joints, tendons and muscles will be subject to variable stresses while generating bodily motion or sustaining impact. There is a constant component of stress due to body weight, a cyclic component from regular movements such as walking and a shock component due to occasional severe loads from jumping or impact. The surface of synovial cartilage is also subject to a tangential shear stress from the relative movement within the synovial joint.

2.2.2 *The chemical environment*

The chemical environment relates to parameters such as; the prevailing medium (gas, aqueous, non-aqueous), the acidity of the medium and the types of dissolved species within the medium. In a similar manner to the physical environment, the chemical environment within the human body is largely uniform but with some critical exceptions. The water content of the body is approximately 60% by weight. Of this 60%, 24% of the body weight is distributed in extracellular fluids such as plasma, interstitial fluids, Lymphatic and transcellular fluids while the remaining 36 % is distributed as intracellular fluids in muscle, bone, connective tissues, red blood cells and others. The function of intracellular fluids is mainly intended for transport of nutrients for life maintaining reactions while the extracellular fluids have multitude of functions including transport of supplies, wastes etc. by plasma, cerebrospinal, lymphatic or urinary fluids and initial digestion of food by gastric secretions, which contain a high concentration of hydrochloric acid.

Water is not present in pure form; instead it is present as aqueous saline solution with dissolved or suspended proteins. The saline solution consists of sodium chloride plus salts of potassium, calcium, magnesium and traces of other metals. The bulk of the metal salts are chlorides but with lesser amounts of carbonate and traces of phosphates and sulfates. Hydrogen is the most common element in the human body by number of atoms (as opposed to atomic mass) followed by carbon and then oxygen. Collectively, carbon, hydrogen, oxygen and nitrogen comprise more than 99% of the human body. Other chemical elements such as calcium, sodium, potassium, phosphorus, sulphur, chlorine, magnesium and iron are present in only small quantities. However small the concentrations of these latter elements are, they still fulfill vital functions as exemplified by the role of iron in blood.

In addition to salts, the dissolved substances present in body fluids include glucose, amino acids, lipids, cholesterol, urea, uric acid and creatinine. The concentrations of these dissolved species vary significantly between blood plasma, cerebrospinal fluid, synovial fluid, pleural and pericardial, peritoneal and any other tissue fluid. The blood plasma contains proteins such as albumin, the globulins, and fibrinogen while haemoglobin is enclosed in erythrocytes (red blood cells). The molecular weight of these proteins ranges from approximately 64,450 for haemoglobin to 340,000 for fibrinogen. As is discussed below, aqueous proteins have a chemical function as well as more specialized physiological functions.

The acidity of most tissue fluids is very moderate with a near neutral pH, i.e. close to pH 7. For example, arterial plasma has a pH of 7.4 while venous plasma has a slightly lower pH due to dissolved carbon dioxide. The body shows a poor tolerance to variations in plasma pH outside of a range of 0.05pH. Outside of the tissues, but still within the body, much larger variations in pH may occur. The contents of the stomach may reach a pH close to 1 during digestion through the secretion of hydrochloric acid. The strong acidity inside the stomach is necessary for the initial digestion of food and to kill any bacteria and viruses ingested with the food. To protect the stomach walls from damage by the hydrochloric acid, the stomach walls are covered with a layer of probably alkaline mucus. Freshly secreted saliva is slightly alkaline; reaching pH 8 and most mucus has an alkaline characteristic. Urine displays considerable variation in pH, ranging from 8 (slightly alkaline) to 4.5 (moderately acidic).

The plasma contains numerous buffers to maintain pH within very narrow limits. A buffer (in a chemical context) is a weak acid or weak base, which has a characteristic pH that is determined by the dissociation constant of the buffer. Dissociation constant is the factor controlling equilibrium between acid (or base) ions and unchanged molecules of acid (or base). Buffers for blood include haemoglobin, other proteins and carbonic acid (dissolved carbon dioxide). Haemoglobin is a very effective buffer since it functions both under acidic and alkaline conditions and because there are numerous dissociation sites on the haemoglobin molecule. Haemoglobin also serves as an aid increasing the oxygen carrying capacity of blood. Oxygen supply to tissues is important to retain the functionality and a human adult requires approximately 250 ml/min of oxygen for oxidizing foodstuffs and produce the energy required for the basic physical well-being. The presence of 150 gms/litre of haemoglobin in blood increases oxygen carrying capacity to 200 ml/litre. This amount of protein in the blood would make blood viscous thus requiring more energy for transport. The carriage of haemoglobins by red blood cells, which occupy about 45% of volume in blood, avoids this rise in viscosity [Brownie and Kernohan, 1999]. Moreover, the haemoglobin solubility is very high in proteins and so the viscosity of blood is not very high compared to the plasma. Tissue fluids other than blood also contain buffers, intra-cellular fluid containing phosphoric acid and proteins as buffers. Interstitial fluids between cells only have carbonic acid as a buffer. Phosphoric and carbonic acids buffer cerebrospinal fluid and urine.

2.2.3   *Changes that occur in pH*

The pH of blood changes with the functions of the body. The respiratory patterns change the pH in blood and cause it to increase or decrease depending on increased rate and depth of breathing or decreased rate and depth of breathing. These are termed as hyper and hypo ventilation. Similar fluctuations in pH can be caused by urinary excretions leading to a condition of Acidosis and Alkalosis depending on the decrease or increase in the pH of blood. Alkalosis or Acidosis is also caused by changes in the metabolic activities. Excessive dosage of aspirin, or caffeine drinks, stress due to exercise or similar activities, uncontrolled diabetes mellitus and diarrhea can cause acidosis in the body while administration of bicarbonate can lead to alkalosis in blood. Associated changes do occur during administration of drugs and a typical example is antibiotics, which decrease the blood pH. Normal treatment of alkalosis includes administration of CO_2 while for acidosis bicarbonate is administered. The ratio of HCO_3 to H_2CO_3 should be maintained at 20:1 to attain the correct pH levels.

2.3 Human cells and cellular matrices

The structure of the body is composed of cells, extra-cellular matrices and tissue fluids. There are a wide variety of cells in the human body, ranging from non-specialized cells that are used to generate new tissue, to specialized cells such as nerve cells. Non-specialized human cells are typically around 10 micrometres in diameter; specialized cells such as muscle or nerve cells grow to a much larger lengths. Specialized cells can adopt almost any shape, from the branched shape of a nerve cell to the tile-like shape of a skin cell. Some cells such as in the skin have a major structural or mechanical function and remain largely in one location. Other cells, such as phagocytes (originating from the immune system with the function of destroying hostile cells and viruses) are much more active and mobile. Phagocytes, either the polymorphs or the macrophages are produced by stem cells that are found in the highest concentration in the bone marrow. The phagocytes therefore have to move from the bone marrow to the site of infection.

Extra-cellular matrices are material that surrounds a cell, usually for structural purposes. A structured extra-cellular matrix is a vital component of tissue since it enables cells to link in regular arrays. Without the matrix, cells are unable to form a coherent structure of linked cells. Bone and cartilage are examples of tissue with large extra-cellular matrices where a network of collagen fibres generate a mechanically strong structure. The proportions of cellular material and extra-cellular matrix vary widely between different tissues; neural tissue has a lower fraction of extra-cellular matrix than bone and cartilage.

2.3.1 *White blood cells*

White blood cells (leukocytes) form a major component of the body's immune system and will probably interact with an implant soon after its placement in the body. White blood cells are formed in the bone marrow where unspecialized stem cells develop in the various specialized types of white blood cell. The diversity of white blood cells enables the body to defend itself against the wide range of pathogens found in nature. A pathogen is any microorganism or organism that is the direct cause of a disease. White blood cell types of particular concern to biomedical implantation are tissue macrophages and neutrophils. Neutrophils are the most common type of white blood cell and have the function of attacking bacteria. Tissue macrophages are much less common than neutrophils and can be considered as auxiliaries (helpers) to the neutrophils. Tissue macrophages tend to form localized complexes around sites of infection or inflammation while neutrophils are more widely distributed.

Neutrophils are attracted to the site of tissue inflammation by sensing the concentration gradients of chemical species released from the inflamed tissues (chemotaxis). Once the neutrophils make contact with the bacteria at the site of inflammation, the neutrophils proceed to either phagocytose (swallow and destroy) the bacteria or kill the bacteria by the release of strong oxidants. Two enzymes found in the neutrophils, NADPH oxidase and Superoxide dismutase generate O_2^- and hydrogen peroxide respectively (Superoxide dismutase uses O_2^- to synthesize hydrogen peroxide). Neutrophils release another enzyme, myeloperoxidase, which converts chloride ions to hypochlorite ions. Myeloperoxidase can also oxidize e.g., bromide ions to hypobromite ions, but the relative abundance of chloride ions in tissue fluids make hypochlorite the main product. These oxidants react with the contents of the bacterial cells to effectively kill the bacteria. It is relevant to note that strong oxidants such as hypochlorite are used in common disinfectants.

While the neutrophils perform a vital role in eliminating bacteria, the patient may experience difficulties when the same chemical response is directed at an implant that has caused inflammation of adjacent tissues. The role of the neutrophils in the immune system is further discussed in Chapter 3 while inflammation problems around implants are discussed in Chapter 4.

2.4 Tissue fluids and circulation systems

There are several different fluids within the body, blood (consisting of plasma and blood cells), the cerebro-spinal fluid (around the brain and spinal cord), pleural fluid (around the lungs), synovial fluid (around the joints), the lymph and digestive secretions, and tears from the eyes. The blood and the lymph have a high cellular content and plasma proteins, approximately 35% by weight for blood. Cerebro-spinal fluid and synovial fluid have much lower concentrations of cells and plasma proteins. The blood is the primary circulation system of the body bringing the necessary nutrients which include minerals, glucose oxygen etc., while the lymphatic fluids collect the waste excreted from the cells as well as fluid that has escaped from the capillaries. The lymphatic system also contains lymph nodes where lymphocytes reside with the purpose of destroying bacteria, viruses, cancer cells and foreign particulate matter.

Plasma proteins have several critical functions such as transport of nutrients, buffering (haemoglobin), maintenance of osmotic pressure, immunity, enzymatic and blood clotting. Liver is the main source for the synthesis of many plasma proteins including albumin, globulins lipoproteins and proteins for blood coagulation.

Besides the transport of erythrocytes (red-blood cells) and dissolved nutrients to the tissues, a major function of blood is the efficient transport of heat via convection since human tissue is a poor conductor of heat. Chapter 4 gives the typical values of conductivity for tissue. An efficient blood circulation is essential for maintaining a uniform temperature in the body since otherwise temperature variations would develop due to external heat loss and metabolic activity within the body. An undesirable side effect of blood circulation is that toxic substances released by a biomedical implant will be rapidly distributed over the whole body.

The CSF (cerebro-spinal fluid) surrounds the spine and brain and facilitates what is termed 'the blood-brain barrier'. Neurons of the brain and spinal cord are protected from exposure to many harmful substances and cells by the "blood brain barrier", interposed between the blood and the CSF by the endothelial cells of the capillaries and the choroid plexus. The CSF also provides a hydraulic cushion to protect the brain from mechanical shock. While characterized by a lower level of metabolic activity than blood, cerebro-spinal fluid is active in the transport of hormones to and from the brain and the control of cerebral blood flow. The CSF is formed in the lateral ventricles, circulates through the interventricular foramens into the subarachnoid spaces, where it diffuses over the brain and spinal cord. It has been calculated that 430 to 450 ml of CSF are produced every day, so the fluid is changed every 6 to 7 hours. Respiratory and circulatory changes are believed to change the pressure within the closed system and promote the mixing and diffusion of fluid.

The synovial fluid is a highly specialized fluid that performs several functions, such as lubricant, cartilage cell nutrient and scavenger of cartilage debris. It is discussed more in detail in chapter 4. The volume of synovial fluid is much less than the volume of almost any other fluid in the human body.

2.5 Summary

The physiological environment in the human body consists of various elements namely, physical and chemical environments, cells and cellular matrices and tissue fluids and circulation systems. The physical and chemical environments in the body are interrelated and change in physical environment affects the chemical environment. The chemical environment within the body is controlled by the body fluids, which are located either inside tissue cells (intracellular fluid) or outside tissue cells (extracellular fluid). There are numerous types of cells, some of which are very likely to interact with an implant, e.g. the phagocytes of the immune system. The various body fluids differ significantly in composition and physical properties such as viscosity.

References

William F. Ganong. *Review of Medical Physiology*, 19th edition, 1999, publ., Appleton and Lange (Simon and Schuster), Stamford, Connecticut, USA.

A.J. Wander, J.H. Sherman, D.S. Luciano, *Human Physiology*, 4th edition, publ., Mc-Graw Hill, New York, 1986.

E.N. Marieb, *Human Anatomy and Physiology*, publ.. Benjamin-Cummings, California, 1989.

University of Akron, General, organic and biochemistry course material. http://ull.chemistry.uakron.edu/genobc/Chapter_25/.

Alexander C Brownie and John C Kernohan, *BIOCHEMISTRY A core text with self assessment*, Churchhill's mastery of medicine, Edinburgh, 1999.

Chapter 3

Implantation and Physiological Responses to Biomaterials

3.1 Introduction

The moment that an implant is placed in the body, there will be a response from the body. Most biomedical materials are so chosen that this response will be favorable. Many other materials initiate a hostile response, which can either cause discomfort to the patient or can seriously affect their health. An example of the former is the soreness caused by the presence of a small wood splinter in the hand. An example of the latter is the blockage of blood vessels by large wear debris from a cardiac implant.

The initial response to an implant resembles the response to a wound since a surgical incision is usually required. Once the initial shock of implantation has passed, there will be a long-term response by the body that may be quite different from the healing of a wound. Careful management of both the initial response and the long-term response to an implant is necessary, if an improvement in the patient's well-being is to be attained.

3.2 Toxic action of implanted materials

An implanted material can become a source of toxicity to the body if an inappropriate material is chosen. As discussed in Chapter 2, human tissue fluids contain numerous salts, proteins and lipids as well as water. A material can either be dissolved by the aqueous fraction of tissue fluids or by the organic fraction. Metals are commonly dissolved by the aqueous fraction with the dissolved salts providing a source of chloride ions to facilitate aqueous corrosion. A common example of a toxic metal is aluminium and its alloys where the trivalent aluminium cation is disruptive to the human metabolism. There have been concerns over the presence of aluminium and vanadium ions. Reduced bone growth and or mineralization have been found in implants containing aluminium and vanadium, the ions of these elements are thought to be possibly implicated [Larsson et al., 2001]. Similarly though the bone is composed of calcium and phosphorous, the concentration of these elements is finely controlled in body fluids such as plasma and cytoplasm of cells. A benign metal such as iron, which is present in haemoglobin, may become toxic if released in excessive quantities by an implant. With the exception of calcium and to a lesser extent iron, the body only requires minute quantities of metals such as cobalt (to form vitamin B12) [Ganong, 1999], zinc, copper, chromium, selenium and magnesium (in larger quantities than the fore-mentioned metals). Most other metals such as lead are toxic to the body because the body has not found a useful role for them in its metabolism.   The body also requires the non-metals, iodine and phosphorous (Phosphorous is from a different family of elements than the halogens which are, fluorine, chlorine, bromine and iodine [Ganong, 1999]. The daily intake of these elements is of the order of 0.1 to 0.01 g with the exception of calcium and phosphorous (approximately 1 g) and magnesium (approximately 0.25g) [Ganong, 1999]. 0.1 to 0.01 g is a very small quantity of metal and it is evident that a large implant containing elements other than calcium, phosphorus and magnesium can easily lead to over-saturation of the body with any given metal if the implant degrades too rapidly. It is also found that concentrations of metal ions of e.g., silver, copper and palladium that are too low to be considered toxic, can significantly affect the functioning of the human immune system [Lewis et al., 2002]. Silver was found to inhibit the activation of immune system monocytes while palladium and to a lesser extent, copper, activated the same cells. It may be concluded therefore that the body is extremely sensitive to the presence of solubilized metals.

Polymers can also be solubilized by the aqueous or organic fraction of tissue fluids; an example is the dialysis tubing that is made from polymers. While the bulk of the polymer may be resistant to solubilization, additives within the polymers such as catalysts and anti-oxidants may be more easily released. Usually these polymer additives can be toxic in a comparable manner to dissolved metals. Polymers are also easily degraded by heat, and sterilization methods involving heat may release toxic degradation products. Kidney dialysis tubing is a common example of this problem.

3.2.1 *Adsorption of toxic substances through the digestive tract*

Most biomaterials for internal use are implanted directly into a body part where there is no direct relationship to the digestive tract. Adsorption of toxic materials via the digestive tract is therefore of limited relevance, however some polymeric materials are used for endoscopic probes and for enteral feeding tubes. The extreme variations in pH and abrasion by digested food particles may cause significant leaching of the polymeric material. Even if the polymer itself is resistant to leaching, minor components of the material such as residual catalysts, processing aids, traces of the original monomer, fillers and anti-oxidants may escape into the digestive tract [Gott, 1997]. With recent developments in autonomous endoscopes that are fitted with cameras, it is conceivable that leaching from the glass and metal of camera lenses and securing rings may become a significant source of inorganic contaminants. A vital feature of the digestive tract, in particular the intestines, is a limiting molecular weight of molecules that pass through the intestinal wall. It appears that substances with a molecular weight greater than 300 Daltons have only limited permeability through the intestinal wall [Gott, 1997]. At higher levels of molecular weight, there is a limited amount of adsorption until 1000 Daltons is reached [Gott, 1997]. Most engineering polymers have molecular weights considerably in excess of 1000 Daltons. Adsorption of toxic substances is not the only cause of risk, a biomaterial in the digestive tract may function as a protected niche for the growth of pathogenic bacteria such as salmonella as is discussed below. Degradation of a biomaterial by enteric bacteria may also generate toxic waste products.

3.2.2 *Initiation of cancer and allergic response to biomaterials*

3.2.2.1 <u>Cancer</u>

The incidence of cancer is most commonly associated with organic chemicals, radiation and viruses. Exposure to inorganic materials such as; cadmium, cobalt, lead and nickel is also associated with cancer [Nowak and Handford, 2004]. For some types of implant involving artificial biomaterials, e.g., orthopaedic implants, the issue of cancer remains a concern [Amstutz and Grigoris, 1996]. A major concern is whether cancer is promoted adjacent to the implant or elsewhere in the body. These concerns about cancer and biomaterials are illustrated schematically in Figure 3.1 Given the concerns about the potential cancer risk of any new biomaterial; it is widely recommended that tests involving cultures of live cells and experimental animals (e.g. rabbits or dogs) should be performed with model implants of the new biomaterial.

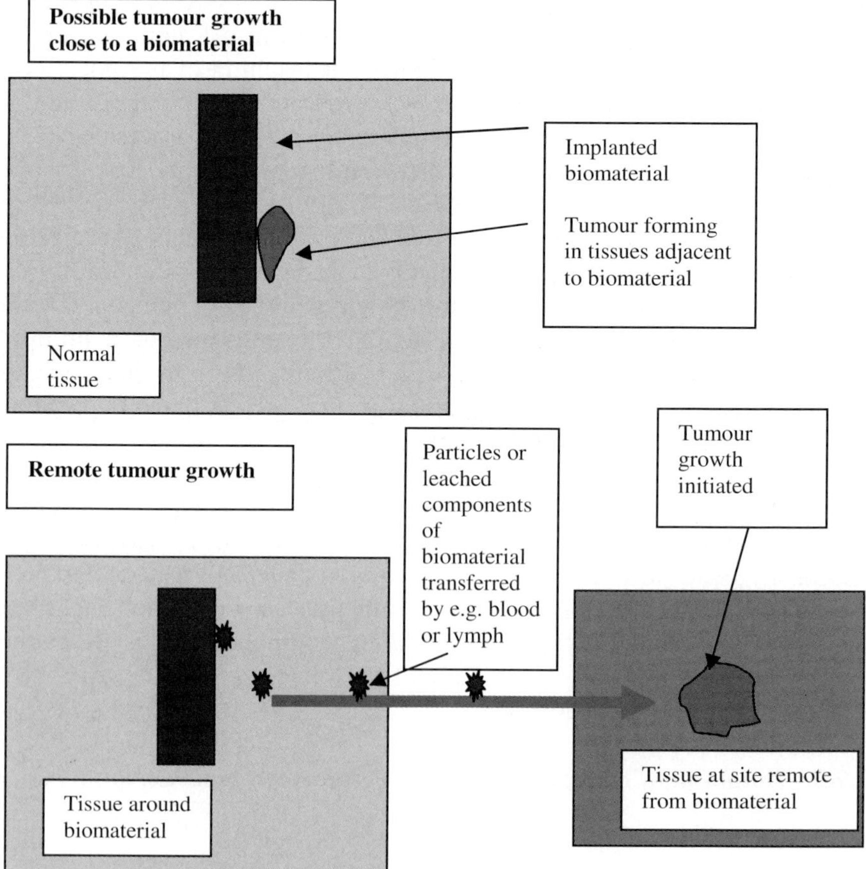

Fig 3.1. Model of possible cancer sites around implanted biomaterials.

Cancer is the uncontrolled growth (increase in number) of abnormal or malignant cells, which eventually reach sufficient number of cells to disrupt the function of a vital organ such as the lung. In normal cells, cellular growth is carefully controlled with a precise balance between destruction of defunct cells and their replacement with new cells.

The most visible sign of cancer is the development of a malignant tumour, which grows until it damages vital organs causing the early demise of the patient. Some tumours, known as benign tumours remain small and effectively isolated from the rest of the body. These benign tumours are relatively harmless compared to the malignant tumours. Tumour growth is however, only the final part of a complex multi-stage process, most biomaterials and implants may become involved with much earlier stages in the disease.

The key stages of cancer are the activation of cells in a given human tissue, e.g. the stomach wall, the initiation of cancer within a group of cells, their promotion or preferential growth over other cells in the presence of carcinogens and finally a change or metastasis to unrestricted growth. Activation is a process where carcinogens (e.g., a complex organic compound) manage to evade cellular defences and reach the cell nucleus to damage the DNA within. If the damaged DNA is not subsequently repaired, as it usually is, daughter cells of the original activated cell will carry a mutated gene. Some, but not all, of these mutated genes may be capable of affecting the cell. The precise mutation that occurs will determine whether or not the affected cell becomes prone to uncontrolled self-replication, or invulnerable to the complex reactions of apoptosis (death of the cell, usually at its own initiation). If the cell has been thus modified, then the cancer process has been initiated. An initiated cell grows more rapidly than normal cells in the presence of foreign substances known as *promoters*. A common example of a promoter is the hydrocarbons found in smoke. A biomaterial could conceivably act as a promoter after implantation. The level of harmfulness of each type of promoter varies with type of human tissue. A biomaterial may therefore become associated with cancer in one type of tissue but not with another tissue type.

At this stage, i.e., promotion, the number of affected cells remains relatively small, with cellular growth only being accelerated during contact with the promoter. A consequence of rapid replication in the presence of a promoter is that the chances of genetic mutation increase significantly. If there is a mutation, which removes the normal control on cellular growth, then the cancerous cells are able to continue growing rapidly without the continued presence of a promoter. The cells start to grow rapidly, i.e. proliferate, and form what is termed a neoplasm (a new growth). If the body is able to encapsulate and isolate the neoplasm (a benign tumor), then the chances of patient survival are much higher. If the neoplasm remains unenclosed and is able to export cancerous cells to other parts of the body (a malignant tumor) then the patient's life is threatened. The transfer or movement of cancerous cells to other parts of the body is known as metastasis. The body's main defence at this stage is a strong immune system, where a form of lymphocyte known as Killer T cells actively source and destroy cancerous cells. A general review of the pathology of cancer and its control by the immune system may be found in discussions of pathophysiology e.g., [Nowak and Handford, 2004].

3.2.2.2   Allergy

Allergy can be loosely defined as an over-reaction by the body to a seemingly harmless substance. A common example of allergy is hay fever, which may require medication for many sufferers. A more serious example of allergy is an intolerance of blood-borne substances such as antibiotics (e.g. penicillin) or the venom of a bee-sting. Blood-borne substances may engender a response by the body known as *anaphylaxis* or anaphylactic shock. Anaphylaxis means anti-protective or destructive while its converse, *prophylaxis* means protective. Anaphylaxis occurs when the immune system is activated to exert a harmful effect on the body. In severe cases, anaphylaxis may cause patient death, often with little time for protective measures to be initiated. A typical fatal complication of anaphylaxis is the expansion of the epiglottis and blockage of the airways to prevent breathing. Some of the typical allergen responses include hay fever, hives, joint pains, asthma, and eczema. Allergies due to materials can be classified into three categories, namely, 1) allergies caused by implants mainly due to immuno-rejection, 2) allergies caused by contact with skin such as jewelry or use of soaps and shampoo etc and 3) Occupational allergy caused due to exposure to elements. Arshad provides a comprehensive description of allergy, its mechanism and consequences [Arshad, 2002].

3.2.2.2.1 *Mechanism of allergies and their classification*

The initiation and mode of allergy is largely controlled by the immune system of the body. A fundamental component of the immune system are antibodies, so called because they attach themselves to and help neutralize foreign 'bodies' such as bacterial cells. Anti-bodies are composed of a specific class of proteins known as immuno-globulins. Immunoglobulins have Y-shaped molecules, which facilitate the attachment of immunoglobulins to either foreign bodies or the cells of the immune system. There are several types of immunoglobulins, IgG, IgM, IgD, IgA and IgE where Ig denotes immuno-globulin. Each type of immunoglobulin is present in differing concentrations in the human serum and has different functions. For instance, IgM initiates a delayed but strong response to bacterial infection while IgG is normally present in the highest concentrations in the blood. IgE is associated with a response to large parasites such as worms in the digestive tract, which can only be expelled by vomiting, diarrhea or sneezing. IgE functions by reacting with its specific allergen (substance causing allergy) on the surface of the mast-cells. The mast-cells then release histamines, heparin, enzymes and tumour-necrosis factor, which initiate the symptoms of allergy. The allergic response that is initiated by IgE is capable of causing anaphylaxis. Blood-borne allergens are particularly dangerous because mast-cells in a variety of bodily locations are activated, not just in a localized site such as the nose or the digestive tract. Implantation of biomaterials will very likely place the biomaterial in close contact with blood vessels.

There are several forms of allergy or hypersensitivity, some involving immunoglobulins other than IgE and some directly involving the cells of the immune system. One form of hypersensitivity that is known to involve dissolved metal ions such as nickel and chromate ions is called delayed-type hypersensitivity [Parham, 2000]. A mitigating feature of this type of hypersensitivity is that the amount of allergen required is much greater than when IgE or another immunoglobulin is involved. The metal ions are chelated (passively react with) by histidine (a component of human proteins). Histidine is then taken up by T-cells from the lymph nodes to initiate an immune response. Figure 3.2 illustrates schematically the significance of allergic response to biomaterials.

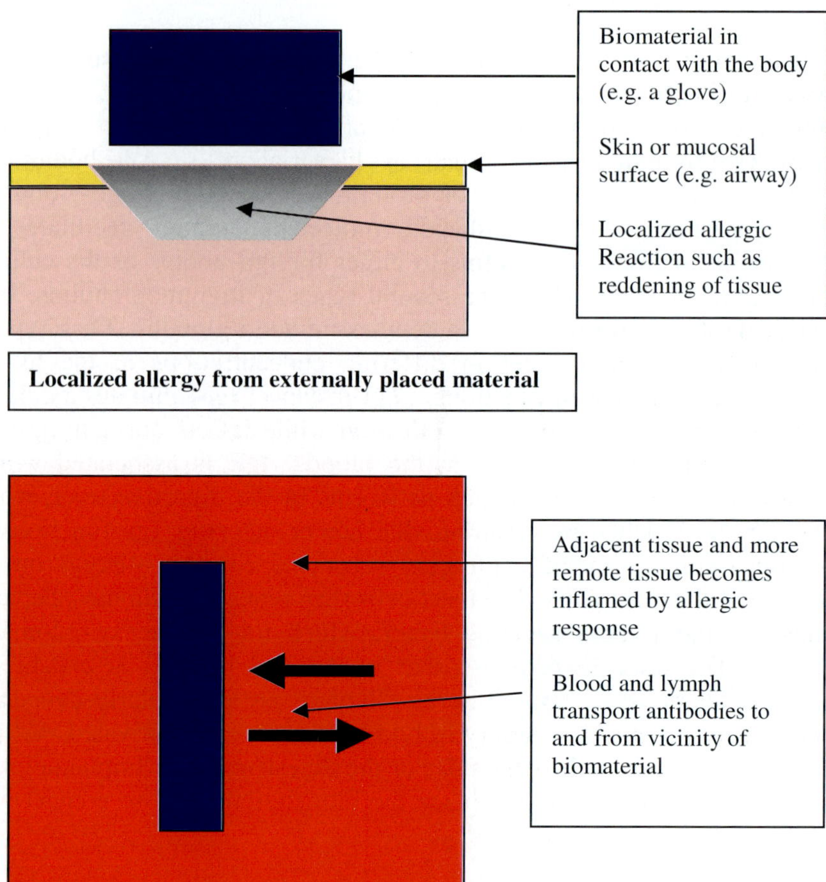

Fig 3.2. Relationship between allergy and biomaterials.

3.2.2.2.2　*Practical causes of allergy*

There are many possible causes of allergy and in many cases; detailed investigation is required to find the specific allergen and the manner in which it reaches the human body. So far as biomaterials are concerned, allergies may arise from a wide range of circumstances.

3.2.2.2.3　*Allergies caused by implants*

These are triggering of allergens by different implants inside the body. While most materials in final product form (implant shape) are not known to cause any allergic responses, the working environment and corrosion trigger allergens to be active. One typical example of such type of allergy is the elution of Aluminium and Vanadium ions and generation of wear particles in case of implants such as dental, artificial stents or joint replacements. Typically the heart implants such as artificial stents are expected to be free from wear but are subjected to erosive wear during transport of fluids. The wear particles thus generated are deposited in other parts of the body, which activates allergens at those sites. Besides wear the hypersensitivity to a particular element also causes allergic responses in patients. Example of such response is amalgams, which use mercury. Mercury is often used as amalgams in dental fillings. Besides being highly toxic, it induces allergic responses such as oral lesions in patients [Pang and Freeman, 1995]. Besides this mercury also causes chronic fatigue syndrome in patients who are hypersensitive to mercury. Nickel another frequently used material in orthodontic implants and jewelry also triggers allergens.

3.2.2.2.4　*Allergies caused by contact*

Allergies caused by casual contact with particular element falls under this category. Ornaments and cosmetics fall in this category, which include jewelry and cosmetic chemicals respectively. Most of the allergic reactions are limited to skin in case of cosmetics and jewelry while implants induced allergies cause further complications besides skin rash. Most common allergy caused by nickel is the dermatitis. Besides nickel causing allergic responses in skin it can trigger off asthma in case of exposure to nickel in occupation.

3.2.2.2.5 *Allergies caused by Occupation*

The allergic responses are also triggered by occupation such as those caused by exposure to fine powders and fibres. Occupational exposure to elements such as nickel, vanadium, and asbestos can cause severe adverse reactions affecting the functions of different organs of the body. Natural latex, but not synthetic latex, contains several different proteins, which are potentially allergenic (i.e. initiating an allergy).   Exposure to natural latex products such as gloves not only may engender an allergic response such as pruritis (itchiness of the skin); but may also increase the difficulty in digesting some common vegetables and fruits, since these contain proteins similar to the proteins found in natural latex [Perkin, 2000].   Latex gloves used by medical professionals and auxiliary staff cause allergic responses that are common in occupation related allergic responses. Latex allergy occurs when the body's immune system becomes sensitized to latex proteins, usually over the course of repeated exposure. As a result of sensitization, the immune system overreacts to latex as a hostile intruder.

Allergic symptoms range from irritating to life threatening, becoming progressively worse with repeated exposure. Allergic symptoms include the following, and may occur singly or in combination:

- Itchy rashes, hives
- Nasal congestion (rhinitis)
- Swelling, especially around the nose, mouth, and throat
- Eye irritation or conjunctivitis
- Respiratory problems, including asthma and rhinoconjunctivitis

Full-blown anaphylaxis, which can include any of the above, can cause death through suffocation or a severe drop in blood pressure.

Allergies are also caused by exposure to asbestos fibres, which leads to a disease called asbestosis or develops cancer. Excessive exposure and inhalation of asbestos fibres causes a buildup of scar-like tissue in the lungs and in the membrane that surrounds the lungs. This scar-like tissue does not expand and contract like normal lung tissue and so breathing becomes difficult. Blood flow to the lung may also be decreased, and this causes the heart to enlarge. This disease is called asbestosis.

Asbestos workers have also an increased risk of getting two principal types of cancer: cancer of the lung tissue itself and mesothelioma, a cancer of the thin membrane that surrounds the lung and other internal organs. Cancer risks are higher for other parts of the body for those who inhale asbestos fibres such as stomach, intestines, pancreas and kidney etc. The cancer in lung tissue may be fatal but the cancers caused in other parts are always fatal.

3.3 Infection from implanted biomaterials

Implantation of biomaterials is associated with significant risks of infection to the patient. There is the risk of contamination during surgery and an impairment of protective immunity by the biomaterial or implant itself [Waldwogel and Bisno, 2000].

3.3.1 *Agents of infection*

A wide range of organisms can cause infection to the human body, these ranges from viruses to bacteria to fungi and protozoa and multi-cellular parasites (e.g. worms). For biomaterials, the most important agent of infection appears to be bacteria. An outline of the salient features of bacteria is given below.

3.3.1.1 <u>Bacteria</u>

Bacteria are single cell organisms lacking a cell nucleus and most other organelles within the cytoplasm (fluid inside the cell). There are a huge variety of bacteria, differing in size, shape and preferred nutrients. Some bacteria are spherical in shape while others are cylindrical; some bacteria require oxygen while others are killed by oxygen. The common characteristic of no cellular nucleus has lead to the classification of bacteria into one group, which is distinct from the other 4 groups that comprise of (1) animals, (2) plants, (3) fungi, (4) protozoa, algae and slime moulds. Bacteria are extremely small, ranging in size from a little more than 100 nm to 10 nm, this small size prevented their discovery until powerful microscopes could be invented. The small size facilitates the rapid entry of nutrients and expulsion of wastes from a cell by diffusion, thus allowing a high metabolic rate and rapid rate of cell division. The lower limit of size of the bacterial cell appears to be controlled by the minimum volume needed to hold a sufficient number of enzyme molecules for effective metabolism. It is estimated that a bacterial cell can hold approximately 1000 enzyme molecules. There is no apparent structure to the cytoplasm (cell contents) apart from a spore, but the cell exterior is made of an inner membrane, a periplasm (liquid around the cell) and a thick cell wall. A spore is spherical body within the cell that functions as a dormant bacterial cell. When the original bacterial cell dies, the spore may survive to regenerate elsewhere. There may also be flagella, projections in the shape of a spiral rod (corkscrew). These flagella give mobility to the bacteria, which can move surprisingly fast compared to their size. Bacterial movement is not random but shows taxis (directed movement) that are controlled by chemical such as a nutrient and physical stimuli such as heat.

Bacteria exist in very large numbers; it is possible for 1,000 billion bacteria to found in a 1 ml sample of water. The small size of the bacteria enables them to have an enormous surface area, the 1,000 billion sample of bacteria can have a combined surface area as high as 3 square metres [Coyne, 1999]. This large surface area greatly facilitates the diffusion of nutrients into bacteria cells and the simultaneous expulsion of their waste products, thus enabling rapid bacterial growth. Bacteria can multiply very rapidly; the salmonella bacteria can double the number of cells within 20 minutes under favorable conditions. A replication rate of doubling every hour means that the bacteria will multiply its number by more than 10 million in 24 hours. When the bacterium reaches this number, it will exert a strong effect on its host (such as a human being). The rapid rate of bacterial replication also presents a major difficulty for the sterilization of implants and any surgical tool. For example, if the said 1,000 billion bacteria are subject to a sterilization process, which leaves only 1 bacterial cell living for every 1 billion killed, i.e., a 1 billion to 1 kill-ratio, there will still remain 1,000 living bacterial cells. Unless the sterilization process is followed either by refrigeration or sufficiently high temperature to prevent regeneration of the bacteria, the bacteria could restore its original number within a few days. In many cases, bacterial growth is limited by the available supply of nutrients and water rather than by sterilization procedures. A dry, non-corroding metal or ceramic surface is likely to control bacterial growth more by deprivation of water and nutrients than by sterilization.

Human beings have to exist surrounded by countless numbers of bacteria, most are harmless or beneficial, such as the enteric bacteria which generate B-group vitamins in the duct. Even if a bacterium does not actively help human life (symbiotic relationship), a bacterial species can still help by depriving pathogenic (disease-causing) bacteria of space and nutrients. Examples of bacteria that commonly live on the outer margins of the human body are Staphylococcus, which is found on the skin and Streptococcus, which is found in the throat. There are two important forms of Staphylococcus, *Staphylococcus albicans* (white coloured), which is essentially harmless and it's more virulent relative *Staphylococcus aureus* (golden coloured), which is discussed below. Both the Staphylococcus and Streptococcus are spherically shaped bacteria of approximately 1 micrometre in diameter.

The relationship between bacteria and the infected person varies greatly between different species of bacteria. In most cases bacteria have evolved so as to feed off their host (a human being) without killing or maiming their host (a host that cannot feed itself will die very quickly along with most of the bacteria living within it). A living host provides an invaluable shelter and source of food for bacteria to proliferate. When the bacteria fail to achieve a benign relationship with the host, illness eventuates. Many bacteria are harmful to human life through their waste products (exotoxins) or through the contents of their cells (endotoxins). Examples of exotoxin release by bacteria are; *Clostridium tetani* (causes tetanus), *Vibrio cholerae* (causes cholera) and *Corynebacterium diptheriae* (causes diptheria) [Parham, 2000]. Endotoxins are usually released when phagocytes engulf bacterial cells [Parham, 2000]. When the bacterial cell disintegrates inside the phagocyte, endotoxins are released that often kill the phagocytes. Since phagocytes are a primary defence mechanism against infection, it can be seen that endotoxins are associated with acute illnesses such as meningitis and typhoid.

Bacteria mostly live extracellularly (i.e., outside of human cells), squeezing into the spaces between cells inside tissue or else floating in body fluids such as blood. Some bacteria however such as the typhoid and plague bacteria live in vesicles inside human cells, which is a form of intracellular existence. It is more difficult for the human body to control intracellular bacterial infections since it may be necessary to sacrifice the infected human cells with consequent damage to tissues and organs.

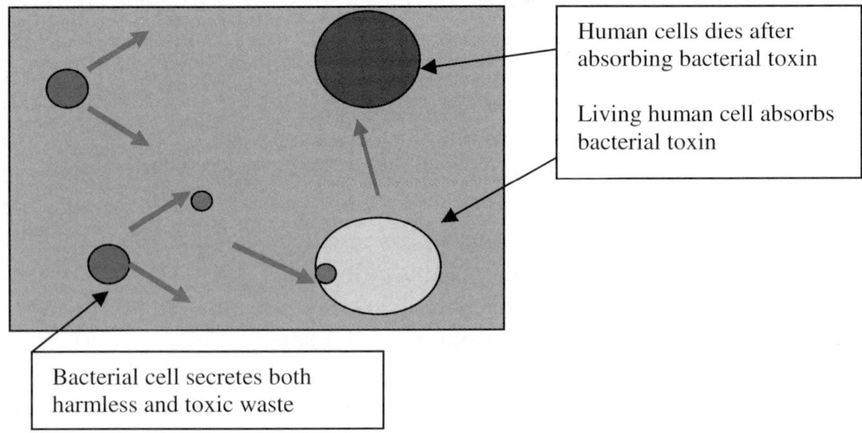

Fig 3.3. Human cell death through absorption of bacterial exotoxins.

The mechanism whereby exotoxins (toxins secreted by bacteria) cause damage to tissues is illustrated schematically in Figure 3.3.

3.3.1.2   Viruses

Viruses are extremely small particles, which cannot be imaged by a light microscope and must infect living organisms before they can transform from a dormant phase to an active phase. Viruses consist of an outer capsule, a core containing a genome of viral DNA or RNA and a conduit, which serves to transfer the viral genome into an infected cell. Being sub-cellular entities, viruses do not contain the enzymes and organelles necessary to operate an active metabolism. This means that, unlike bacteria, which can thrive in an extracellular mode, viruses can only proliferate intracellularly. Viruses replicate by injecting their DNA or RNA into a target cell, where they subvert the biological machinery of the cell so that it produces more virus particles rather than normal cell products. The daughter virus particles are then released from the infected cell to proceed to infect other susceptible cells. To enter a cell, the virus particles must first engage with a surface molecule on the exterior of the cell. The specific receptor to which the virus binds determines which tissues are susceptible to infection. Even in the case of phagocytic cells, a virus must still bind to specific surface molecules.

If many virus units are produced from each infected cell, then an exponential growth in virus number is possible just as is the case with bacterial infections. Many common viruses such as those causing smallpox, chickenpox, measles and hepatitis are pathogenic (cause illness) by direct destruction of the infected cells. Other viruses are pathogenic because of the extreme response generated by the human immune system. In an effort to protect the human body, the immune system can often cause many side effects, leading to illnesses that worsen the original infection. In some cases, e.g., the Epstein-Barr virus infections, the viral DNA can become integrated with the DNA of the host (i.e., the infected person). The Epstein-Barr virus causes infectious mononucleosis as well as some more serious complications [CDC, 2002]. In this clinically quiescent situation, viral DNA persists and is replicated when the host cell divides. Depending on the sites of integration, viral DNA can give rise to mutations of host DNA, indirectly causing a cancerous change.

3.3.2　*Infection from arterial prostheses, prosthetic heart valves, orthopaedic implants, and catheters*

The risk of infection is present for any biomaterial when it is in close contact with the body or body fluids. Prosthetic heart valves, orthopaedic implants and catheters involve entry into parts of the interior of the body where the consequences of infection are very severe for the patient. It is critically important that the biomaterials for these applications and others engender the minimum possible infection risk. The catheter is a relatively small implant compared to e.g. an artificial hip, but if contaminated by bacteria can exert a prolonged and highly detrimental effect on the patient. More elaborate devices with powered systems, such as pacemakers, can also create infection risks for the patient.

3.3.2.1　<u>Arterial prostheses and Prosthetic heart valves</u>

Arterial prostheses and prosthetic heart valves share a common problem of post-operative infection [Goeau-Brissonnier and Coggia, 2000; Karchmer, 2000]. Allowing for late infections as well as infections soon after implantation, the infection rate for arterial prosthesis is a few percent [Goueau-Brissonnier and Coggia, 2000]. Estimates of the infection rate for valve prostheses range from 1 to 9% [Karchmer, 2000], where prosthetic valve endocarditis occurs. For arterial implants, the common cause of infection is a variety of bacteria such as *Staphylococcus epidermis* and *Staphylococcus aureus* with enterobacteria also being a significant source. Fungi may also be involved and the likelihood of a particular microorganism being the source of infection varies significantly with type of arterial implant. The consequences of infection for the patient can be serious and diagnosis may become difficult when there is a late slow infection [Goeau-Brissonnier and Coggia, 2000]. For prosthetic heart valves, Staphylococcus aureus and Staphylococcus epidermis are the major causes of infection together with enteric (from the gut) bacilli (rod-shaped bacteria). However, as with arterial implants, it appears that a wide variety of microorganisms may cause infection if they have been able to contaminate the prosthesis [Karchmer, 2000]. As with arterial implant infections, the consequences of prosthesis infection for the patient are serious with numerous, unpleasant, potential medical complications.

3.3.2.2 Orthopaedic implants

Despite the extremely high level of attention given to sterility in the operating room, some recipients of implants suffer from post-operative infection. With orthopaedic implants, the most common source of such infections is believed to be the operating room where the implantation was performed [Steckelberg and Osmon, 2000]. Infection risks are higher with orthopaedic implants than other comparable implants because of the impaired effectiveness of antibiotics and localized disturbance of the immune response around the implant caused by the generation of wear particles (further discussed in Chapter 4). The action of antibiotics is impeded by the poor vascularity (lack of capillaries close to the synovial joint) and the presence of detritus and necrotic tissue. Osteomyelitis is a typical infection of bony connective tissue caused by bacteria or fungi after implantation. In other words it causes inflammation of bones. The typical microorganisms causing Osteomyelitis are the staphylococci including *Staphylococcus aureus, Pseudomonas aeruginosa* and more rarely, *Escherichia coli.* [Steckelberg & Osmon, 2000]. Staphylococci including *Staphylococcus aureus* form the largest single bacterial source of infections. Other bacteria and even fungi have been found to cause infections in a few cases [Steckelberg and Osmon, 2000]. In most situations the bacteria introduced during trauma and surgery stay dormant for months before it starts invading the body tissues. The effect of such invasion is the inflammatory response and potentially necrosis of tissue. Implanted biomaterial surfaces can provide an environment conducive for bacterial contamination and colonization. However, immediately upon implantation the biomaterial surface is coated with body fluids, which are anionic in nature. This acts as a protective barrier against bacterial invasion since they are also anionic in nature and the body fluid film coating partially repels the colonization of bacteria. If during this stage, the healthy tissue interact with the film the bacteria may be blocked and there may not be an infection. On the other hand if the bacteria interact with the biomaterial surface before the healthy tissue it would lead to undesirable tissue reactions. The initial surface conditions play a vital role on the adhesion of proteins to the implant surface and the thickness of the film decides on the interaction between healthy tissues or bacteria and the biomaterial surface. One of the methods currently practiced include passive coating of surface to promote body fluid film formation (Allan et. al., 2002).

3.3.3 *Infection mechanisms, bacterial biofilms and contaminated catheters*

The surface and in some cases the interior of biomaterials provide an excellent niche for bacteria and fungi. Since most biomaterials are implanted deep within the human body, e.g. orthopaedic implants, the potential for severe infection is very high. *Staphylococcus epidermis*, as mentioned above, is virtually harmless when present on the skin, but can cause a life-threatening infection when it manages to penetrate muscle or internal organs. This means that an implant does not have to be contaminated with an exotic, virulent species of microorganism to present a risk. Common microorganisms such as are carried by water or float in the air, have the potential to cause major difficulties for a patient receiving an implant. The problem of severe infection caused by inadvertent transport of bacteria to deep within the body is illustrated schematically in Figure 3.4.

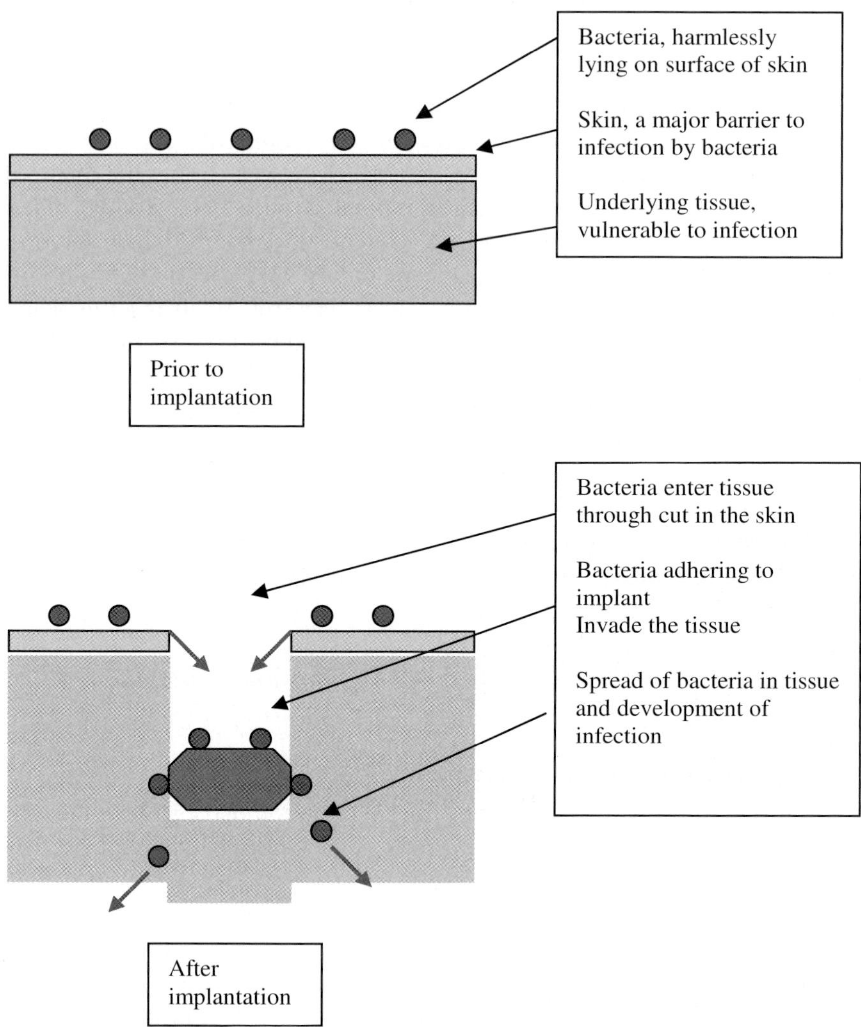

Fig 3.4.   Invasion of bacteria into deep tissue during and after implantation of a biomaterial.

3.3.3.1   Bacterial biofilms

Bacteria are not only present as single cells but can also group together to form colonies or 'biofilms'. As described above, bacterial tend to adhere to fixed surfaces, once a sufficient density of bacterial cells are established on the surface, the bacteria tend to aggregate together in colonies. A process of attraction between adjacent bacterial cells occurs at this stage and it is known as 'quorum sensing' [McCarthy, 2001]. The bacterial cells then begin to accumulate in layers while at the same time developing a communal extra-cellular matrix. This extra-cellular matrix is composed of polysaccharides and effectively protects the bacterial cells against antibiotics and most other bactericidal substances. A further stage of growth occurs where the bacteria form tower-like structures approximately 100 micrometres tall, at this stage most of the colony is composed of extra-cellular matrix. The colony contains channels and ducts to allow nutrients to enter and waste products to be released. There is also considerable differentiation between individual bacterial cells within the colony, with particular functions for each cell. The concept of a biofilm is illustrated schematically in Figure 3.5.

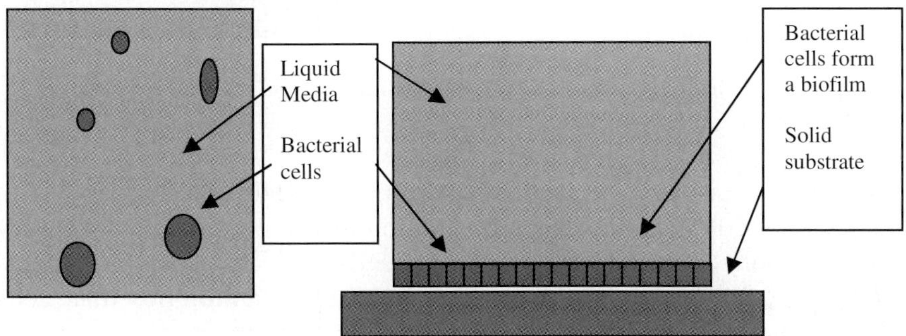

Fig 3.5. Bacteria as isolated free flowing cells and in a biofilm.

Once a bio-film is formed, the constituent bacteria are much more resistant to phagocytosis, which is the body's main response to control bacteria. This resistance would appear to be caused by the inability of the neutrophils and macrophages to detach bacteria from the biofilms prior to phagocytosis. The resistance of biofilms to phagocytosis is illustrated schematically in Figure 3.6.

Biofilms are estimated to be 1,000 times more resistant to common anti-biotics [McCarthy, 2001] and may even secrete enzymes that degrade antibiotics. It should be noted that antibiotics themselves exert toxic effects on the human body and there is a limiting safe dosage. It has been found that the extra-cellular matrix contains these enzymes. The biofilm

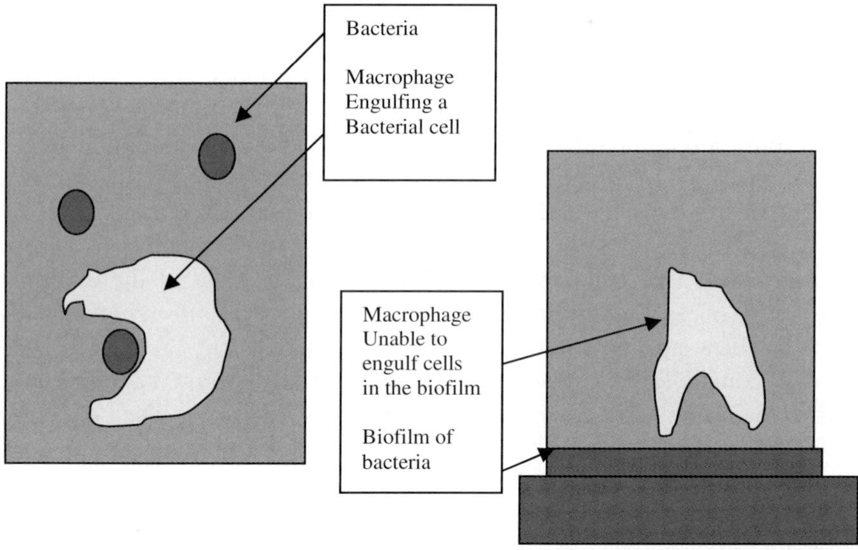

Fig 3.6. Enhanced resistance to phagocytosis by bacteria found in a biofilm.

has another measure to protect itself against antibiotic attack, deep within the bacterial colonies, there is a population of bacterial cells with a very low metabolic rate. These bacterial cells, which resemble spores [McCarthy, 2001, Stewart], are more resistant to antibiotics than cells with a higher metabolic rate.

The study of bacterial biofilms in the human body is a relatively new field that was originally subject to much scepticism [McCarthy, 2001]. It is becoming apparent that biofilms represent a radically different aspect of bacterial life from the traditional concept of individual bacterial cells and spores floating freely in a liquid or gaseous medium.

A critical concern is the spontaneous development of antibiotic resistant bacteria. The most well known example of this is the Methicillin resistant *Staphylococcus Aureus* (MRSA) where Methicillin is an antibiotic. It is very different to eradicate a colony of MRSA once it has formed on a urinary catheter [Jones et al., 2001]. The internal surface of the catheter forms an excellent site for a biofilm of pathogenic bacteria. Biofilm formation in a catheter is illustrated schematically in Figure 3.7.

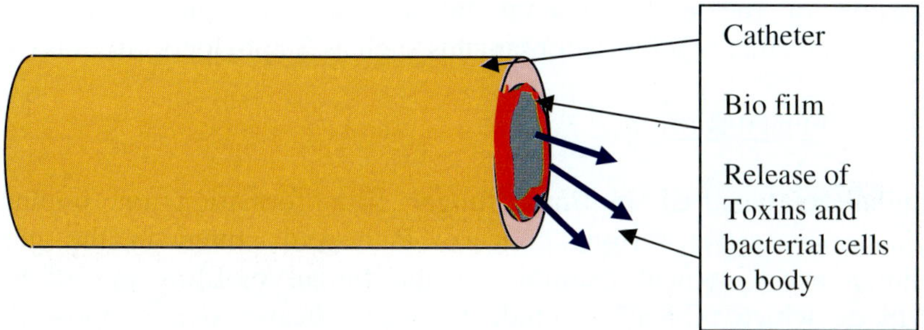

Fig 3.7. Biofilm formation in a catheter by pathogenic bacteria.

In some cases, the biofilm can become thick enough to block flow through a catheter. An important example of this is the blockage of urinary catheters by colonies of *Proteus mirabilis* [Stickler et al., 2003].

Detailed studies have revealed that MRSA are able to develop colonies on a silastic rubber surface even when prophylatic antibiotics such as vancomycin or rifampicin are applied. The formation of biofilms from resistant bacteria such as MRSA on the surfaces of biomaterials is a key issue of concern in the use of implants [Jones et al., 2001]. The virtual impossibility of destroying biofilms once they enter the human body means that almost perfect sterilization and perfectly clean handling of the implant is required prior to implantation in the body.

Another factor, which influences formation of bacterial biofilms, is the substratum properties. The adhesion and colonization of bacterial biofilms differ based on the surface properties and the type of material used. Preferential adhesion takes place depending on whether plastics, metals or glass are used as implants. Typical examples include frequent occurrence of *Staphylococcus epidermidis* colonization in organic polymer surfaces compared to *Staphylococcus aureus* on metallic substrates. In a similar manner, the adherence of *E.coli* and *Klebsiella* is higher with latex and latex-teflon compared to silicone based catheters. The typical surface properties such as surface charge, hydrophilicity – hydrophobicity and texture have influence over the bacterial biofilm adhesion and formation on different implant surfaces. Given the propensity of bacteria to colonize the surface of any implant for later invasion of the body, a vital future research topic is to design biomaterials that repel microorganisms such as Staphylococcus aureus.

3.3.3.2   Fungal Biofilms

Similar to bacterial biofilms fungal film formation on implants/ biomaterials cause serious concern. Pathogenic fungi in the genus candida are a typical example of the fungal biofilms on implants surfaces, which typically include prosthetic heart valve or indwelling catheters. The research on fungal biofilms lags behind the bacterial bio film research. *Candida* spp. is frequently identified as agents of nosocomial pneumonias and urinary tract infections. An implanted device such as an intravascular or urinary catheter, or endotracheal tube, is associated with these infections and a biofilm can be detected on the surface of the device. Other devices totally implanted into the body, such as prosthetic heart valves, cardiac pacemakers and joint replacements (e.g. hip or knee), are also liable to candidal infection, usually at the time of surgical placement.

3.3.3.3   Fever and elevation of body temperature

The human body reacts quickly to the presence of hostile microorganisms by activating the immune system and in some cases releasing agents that promote fever, these are known as pyrogens. An implant which is sensitive to temperature, e.g. contains a thermostatic switch may be inadvertently activated by the body temperature change that is induced by fever. Micro-machines that depend on fine clearances between moving parts may malfunction because of loss of sliding clearance caused by differential thermal expansion.

3.3.3.4   Effect of immediate adsorption of proteins on surface

A surface film of adsorbed proteins will significantly affect the friction and wear characteristics of an implant. Despite their extreme thinness, adsorbed films of almost any chemical species have a profound effect on the friction and wear of most materials. This is because the adsorbed film controls the molecular and electronic exchanges occurring at the sliding contact interface.

Once placed inside the body, any implant requiring mechanical movement will have different functional characteristics. While the effect of protein adsorption is not entirely harmful, there are problems of increased wear and wear-induced pitting corrosion of metals. The effect of protein adsorption on mechanical function is discussed further in Chapter 4, where it is particularly relevant in the specialized context of orthopaedic prostheses.

3.3.3.5   <u>Effect of immune response on biomaterials</u>

As discussed in Chapter 2, tissue inflammation causes neutrophils (a form of white blood cell) to release strong oxidants such as hydrogen peroxide and hypochlorite. Hydrogen peroxide can oxidize iron from the ferrous to the ferric state via the Stanton reaction. The presence of free ferric ions (a chemically active species) in the body would almost certainly be undesirable. Hydrogen peroxide is known to accelerate the wear rate of polymers such as UHMWPE in sliding contact with a hard metal surface. A similar effect may occur with hypochlorites, but so far no published data appears to be available.

3.3.4   *Sterilization of biomaterials*

Given the critical importance of controlling the spread of bacteria and other parasites throughout a biomaterial, sterilization of biomaterials is of vital concern. Despite the advanced nature of modern sterilization technology, it is not possible to be completely assured of sterility in a biomaterial after processing. A criterion to define the quality of sterilization is the Sterility Assurance Limit (SAL), which is the statistical probability that a given implant is non-sterile. The generally accepted value of SAL is 1 in a million [Ratner et al., 1996]. There are now four main methods of sterilization, the traditional immersion in high-pressure steam at approximately 120 degrees Celsius, fumigation of the implant with either pure ethylene oxide or a mixture of ethylene and carbon dioxide, irradiation with gamma-rays from an isotope source and more recently immersion in a super-critical carbon dioxide. High-pressure steam is very effective at destroying bacteria but is also destructive to many of the polymers that are used as biomaterials. This is because 120 degrees Celsius is higher than the glass transition temperature of most polymers. Ethylene oxide is effective and works at room temperatures, the disadvantage is that ethylene oxide is as toxic to human life as it is to bacterial life. This means that the implant must be 'washed' by the passage for several hours of sterilized air to remove any residual ethylene oxide from the implant. There is often an element of doubt whether the biomaterial will react with the ethylene oxide to create a permanently bound toxic residue. Gamma radiation from a Cobalt 60 source is rapid, gives a high quality of sterilization and does not leave any toxic residue [Rose et al. 1984, Gilbertson 1995]. The main limitations of Cobalt 60 sterilization procedures are the high equipment cost, safety risks and effect on the irradiated material (discussed in Chapter 4). A new process employs the unique properties of supercritical fluids, especially of super-critical carbon dioxide. A super-critical fluid is one where the temperature is too high for a vapour to liquefy. Carbon dioxide at ambient temperatures and a pressure of 20 MPa is found to sterilize common infectious bacteria such as Staphylococcus Aureus [Dillow et al. 1999]. Carbon dioxide is believed to kill the bacteria by dissolving inside their cellular cytoplasm and altering the cellular pH (acidity). SFE sterilization involves non-toxic gases and a relatively moderate equipment cost; however it is still not widely used.

3.3.5 *The protective responses of the body*

The human body has evolved a wide range of defences against invading pathogens (agents of disease). There are passive non-specific defences, which are found in the skin, the digestive system and in the respiratory tract. When these prove inadequate, a series of cellular processes known as the immune response is activated. The immune response is effective at eliminating pathogens but exerts a disruptive effect on normal body functioning, thus compounding the loss of well-being that we feel when we become ill.

3.3.5.1   Passive non-specific defenses

The skin contains an outer layer of cells that are toughened by a protein called keratin. The skin is able to physically separate the internal organs of the body from the pathogens outside because of the toughness conferred by keratin and other features of the skin. Any break in the skin caused by a cut or a burn renders the body vulnerable to entry and infection by pathogens. The implantation of most biomaterials necessarily requires penetration of the skin with the attendant risks of infection.

A salient feature of the stomach is the high level of acidity during the digestion of food. This acidity not only decomposes the food but also destroys most bacteria that may be ingested with the food.

The respiratory tract (throat and lungs) and the stomach are covered with a thin film of semi-liquid mucus, where the sticky consistency of mucus is generated by proteins known as mucins. The mucus in the stomach protects the cells of the stomach wall from the severe acidity of the stomach contents. In the respiratory tract, the mucus flows outwards from the interior of the respiratory tract to the nose and mouth. The mucus flow is guided by fine cilial hairs on the surfaces of the respiratory tract. This outward flow of mucous effectively expels bacteria entrained during breathing. The mucus also contains enzymes and proteins that inhibit any infections that may arise.

The saliva of the mouth and the tears in the eyes contain an enzyme known as lysozyme, which is bactericidal (kills bacteria).

3.3.5.2   The immune system and the immune response

The human immune system, which enables us to resist infections, is highly complex, and even today our understanding of it remains incomplete [Batchelor, 2003]. Undoubtedly one reason for this complexity is the sheer variety of potentially damaging agents, which humans may encounter. Thus a response, which may be highly effective against one agent, may be ineffective against another. Natural selection therefore favours the evolution of an immune system with several effector pathways. This almost certainly explains why the human immune response includes soluble protein antibodies of different classes and functions, a variety of white cells with different functions, inter-cell-messenger molecules (cytokines & chemokines), and proteins of the complement system. Another reason for complexity is that appropriate immune responses are needed against frequent, but low severity infections such as bacterial ingress through minor skin abrasions, but also against less common, potentially virulent systemic infections, e.g. measles virus.

A further vital aspect of the immune system is that it should remain tolerant of "self", while maintaining its powers to recognize and react against "non-self" molecules. Maintaining tolerance of "self" is partly achieved by systematic destruction of potentially self-reactive T lymphocytes as they progress through a series of differentiation stages in the thymus. The lymphocyte population that emerges from the thymus is largely purged of dangerous, self-reactive T lymphocytes. However, there are also important and incompletely understood mechanisms of tolerance operating in the peripheral tissues, and there is now persuasive evidence that tolerance is constantly maintained by presentation of self-components to the body's lymphocyte population. Under some circumstances, self-tolerance may fail and result in immunity against the self (auto-immunity). During inflammatory reactions, some leukocytes attracted to the site secrete lymphokines and other chemical messenger molecules that indirectly encourage immunity. Although the evidence remains incomplete, there is a widely held view that persistent inflammation can interfere with maintenance of self-tolerance. From the biomaterials scientist's perspective, it is clearly desirable to avoid using materials for implants that risk inciting either immune or strong inflammatory responses [Batchelor, 2003].

The immune response involves a series of specialized cells found mainly in the lymph glands, the spleen, the thymus and in the blood. These cells constitute the immune system, which has evolved with the purpose of terminating infection by viruses, bacteria, fungi and small multi-cellular parasites (such as worms). As discussed in Chapter 4 in relation to orthopaedic implants, there is no evolutionary precedence for the implantation of biomaterials, which often causes a confused, destructive response by the immune system.

The main cell types, which deliver the immune response, are the leukocytes (white blood cells) and the lymphocytes (cells of the lymph glands). The leukocytes and other cells such as macrophages, destroy invading pathogens by phagocytosis. Phagocytosis is a process where the human cell surrounds and then engulfs a foreign cell or small organism. The macrophages and leukocytes are particularly attracted to cells, which have been coated by antibodies. This is a basic reason why acquired immunity is effective at dealing with repeat infections; the body already contains a stock of primed antibodies to detect and coat the invading bacteria or human cell infected by a virus.　Once the target cell is engulfed, the leukocyte or macrophage releases comparatively large quantities of strong enzymes and oxidants, which destroy the target cell. The process of phagocytosis is illustrated schematically in Figure 3.8.

Phagocytosis also exerts a destructive effect on the human cells too, so the leukocytes and macrophages only have a short life. The gathering of leukocytes and macrophages around an infection site occurs simultaneously with an inflammation of the infected tissues. Inflammation involves localised temperature elevation to accelerate metabolic processes and swelling of the capillaries to enlarge the pores in the walls of the capillaries. This allows the leukocytes to pass through the pores and enter the infected tissue to destroy bacteria. Anti-bodies also pass through the pores of adjacent lymph vessels into the tissue.

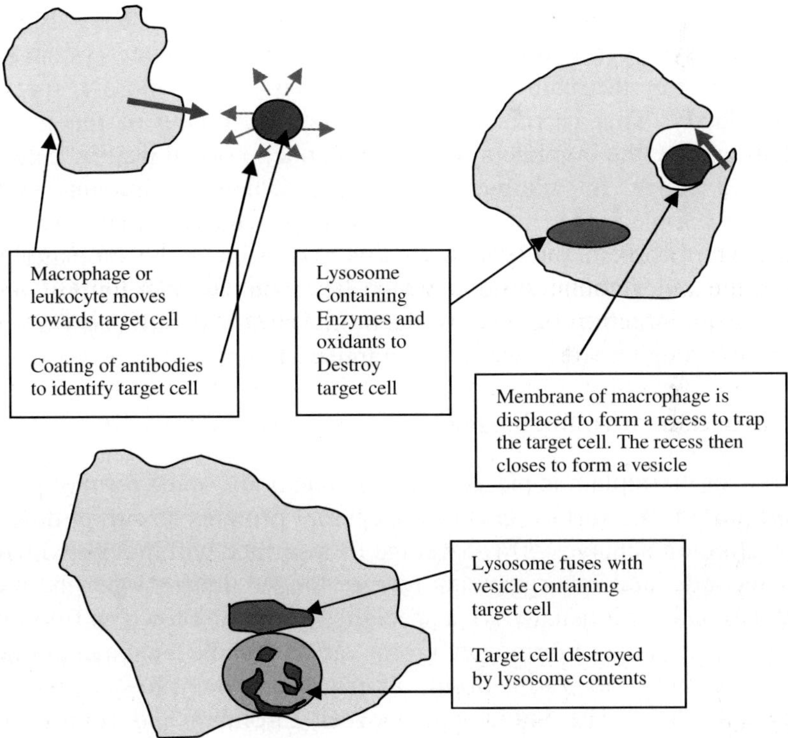

Fig 3.8. Mechanism of phagocytosis where a targeted cell is destroyed.

As described in the discussion on Allergies, anti-bodies are a form of globulin proteins, immunoglobulins, which are present in several different forms, i.e., IgG, IGM, IgA, IgE and IgD. The anti-bodies adhere to molecules of bacterial exotoxin or to the cell walls of bacterial cells. The adherence by antibodies on bacterial cells helps the phagocytes to engulf the exotoxin molecules or bacterial cells. The anti-bodies have a memory characteristic that is specific to an individual microbe or toxin, which is generated by a specialized form of lymphocyte, the B-cells. When there is a repeat infection, the subset of B-cells that carry a record of the earlier infection, are encouraged to multiply rapidly and release the appropriate anti-body. This memory characteristic is greatly superior to the original unspecialized response by the antibodies and is the basis of immunization. Certain parasites, viruses in particular, rapidly mutate (change their genetic code) so that the immunization from an earlier infection is not longer effective.

A highly developed and specialized feature of the immune system is its specificity, i.e. the ability to focus its attack on a closely specified foreign body. This is vital to the smooth functioning of the immune system, or else the immune system could attack normal healthy cells. As discussed above, an allergic attack occurs when the immune system reacts to harmless foreign substances and damages normal tissue as a result. The problem for biomaterials is that even if the biomaterial is innoccuous, i.e. contains no toxic metals (such as aluminium) or no carcinogenic organic compounds, the biomaterial may still cause a health problem through disturbance of the immune system.

3.4 Reactions with fibrinogen

As soon as an implant is placed in the human body, some form of protein absorption on the surface occurs.   Different proteins absorb at different rates, albumin achieves 50% coverage of a surface within approximately 0.05 seconds, and other proteins require longer times. When the tissue fluid is blood (as it usually is), a specialized protein known as fibrinogen becomes activated. Fibrinogen is converted by the enzyme thrombin (also a protein) to form fibrin, which takes the physical form of entangled fibres. The interaction between thrombin and fibrinogen is controlled by an inter-related series of reactions (which is an example of a 'cascade') so that fibrin formation only occurs where it is needed [Marieb, 1989].

Adsorption of proteins such as fibrinogen on the surface of a biomaterial may upset the delicate balance of chemical reactions in the clotting mechanism. Of particular concern is an unpredicted activation of the clotting mechanism close to the implant. Most clots are dismantled by the process of *fibrinolysis*, which is performed by the enzyme *plasmin*. Rapid clot destruction is essential to prevent the eventual clogging of blood vessels by clots since blood vessels are continuously developing leaks. Where a clot survives it is termed a *thrombus* and a thrombus that detaches to float in the blood stream is called an *embolus*. Any embolus can block a blood vessel of smaller diameter, causing severe damage to the surrounding organ such as the heart, lung or brain. Any biomaterial, which increases the risk of thrombus and embolus formation, would be hazardous to the patient.

3.4.1 *Role of plasma proteins and platelets*

The prompt formation of a blood clot to prevent excessive bleeding is the result of a complex multi-stage interaction between platelets and proteins in the blood. As described above, fibrin is a major component of the blood clot (formation of a blood clot is known as *haemostasis*).

Platelets provide a critical early response to blood loss by forming the initial clot. Platelets enclosed by a membrane and contain a cytoplasm like cells, but differ from cells in other respects. Platelets are very small (2 to 4 micrometres in diameter), do not have a nucleus and contain specialized features that facilitate haemostasis. There are a very large number of platelets in the human blood, approximately 250,000 to 500,000 per micro-litre. Each platelet contains a large number of 'granules' and is surrounded by a large number of microtubules. When a blood vessel is cut, platelets are rapidly attracted to the cut by the exposed collagen fibres of the blood vessel. Adhesion of the platelets to collagen is considered to be a passive process (little expenditure of energy) and is only a part of the normal functions of platelets. A process known as *Platelet activation* occurs when platelets bind to collagen or neutrophils and monocytes release the *Platelet Activation Factor* (PAF). Activation of platelets causes them to adhere to contacting tissue and to change shape. Shape changes involve both swelling and the extension of processes (microscopic 'tentacles') for adhesion to the blood vessel. Secretions from the activated platelets cause the cut blood vessel to contract and further restrict blood flow. Platelet activation is a carefully controlled process since haemostasis is harmful when it occurs at sites remote from a leak in a blood vessel. The rapid response of platelets is followed by the deposition of a fibrin network, which binds erythrocytes (red blood cells) to the clot. The larger size of the erythrocytes compared to platelets facilitates the formation of a stronger clot than the original platelet clot.

During normal blood flow, platelets are not attracted to the walls of blood vessels (the endothelium) because of the positive charge on the endothelium. Rupture of the blood vessels exposes the negatively charged collagen fibres. For vascular implants, it would appear desirable to have a positive charge on the surface of the biomaterial and a negative charge inside, in order to prevent adhesion by platelets.

3.5 Cell-biomaterial Interactions

Human cells, being active and mobile, will interact with a biomaterial soon after implantation and the initial absorption of proteins. Non-human cells, e.g. bacterial cells may interact with biomaterials before implantation, this generally causes problems for the patient. Effective management of cell-biomaterial interactions is essential for successful functioning of the implant. Examples of positive cell-biomaterial interactions are growth of bone cells on orthopaedic implants (described in Chapter 4), negative interactions are exemplified by the aggregation of large numbers of white blood cells in the inflamed tissue around an orthopaedic implant.

3.5.1 *Mechanism of cell adhesion*

Many components of human tissue, e.g. lipids show a non-specific adhesion to common artificial materials such as glass [Wang et al. 2000]. This bonding may either involve Van der Waals forces or electrostatic bonding for proteins, which are charge-sensitive [Sittig et al., 1999 (both articles)]. Attachment between adjacent cells in a tissue is controlled by more highly developed forms of adhesion involving proteins such as integrins.

3.5.1.1   Intra-cellular adhesion and the construction of tissue

Human cells display a tendency to adhere to each other and to extra-cellular matrices. Specialized molecules embedded in cell membranes have the purpose of generating adhesion between cells. The adhesion is specific to particular combinations of cells and based partly on interlocking between proteins of contacting cells. The adhesion between cells and with an extra-cellular matrix enables the formation of tissue as opposed to isolated cells. There are four basic classes of proteins necessary for inter-cellular adhesion, laminins, immunoglobulins, cadherins and integrins. The immunoglobulins are part of the immune system and enable white blood cells to function. In cases where a biomaterial is the subject of hostile response by the immune system, these cellular adhesion proteins would play a significant but as yet poorly understood role. The inter-cellular adhesion proteins also transmit signals between cells, a condition that is found to be necessary for the normal functioning of human cells.

3.5.1.2 Adhesion to alien materials

The adhesion of human cells to implanted biomaterials varies widely with materials. Many metals are toxic and the cells are unable to remain in close contact with the metals. Instead, a thin necrotic or inactive layer a few micrometres thick is formed between the cells and the implant. Aluminium is a clear example of localised necrosis, as discussed above. Only a weak adhesion is achieved for these materials. This characteristic of poor adhesion is relevant to dressings containing paraffin gauze with thin metallic aluminium gauze for preventing adherence.

Other metals, e.g., titanium, are virtually non-toxic to tissue and adhesion usually occurs. Titanium is widely used as an orthopaedic or dental implant because human cells such as osteoblasts strongly adhere to this metal [Sittig et al. 1999]. Titanium is usually covered by an oxide film, the various proteins of the body readily absorb to the oxide film. If titanium or other metals are not covered by an oxide film, e.g. after cutting, the nascent metal surface produced would be very reactive and may decompose proteins or other biochemicals. It is also found that the composition of the oxide film is modified after protein adsorption. Adhesion of proteins and cells to titanium is the subject of current research [Spencer 2002, Kenausis et al. 2000, Huang et al., 2001].

A third class of materials, the *bioactive materials* (discussed further in Chapter 4) demonstrate an entirely different response. Cells, particularly those with an extra-cellular matrix that is related to the material, grow in close contact with the material to obliterate the boundary between implant and tissue. With such bioactive materials, a high level of adhesion is obtained. In other cases where there is no *bio-activity*, it would be expected that proteins, which absorb on both metals and cell membranes, function as a form of 'adhesive'.

3.5.1.3 Detrimental adhesion by bacterial cells

Strong cellular adhesion is not entirely beneficial, bacterial cells are able to bind to extra-cellular proteins such as fibrinogen, fibronectin and to collagens, thereby generating infection sites in the body [Ross]. If bacterial cells display strong adhesion to biomaterials, forming *biofilms*, implantation of the biomaterial into the patient would probably cause severe infection. Bacterial contamination has been cited as a major risk for cardiac implants [Ross]. Adhesion by the bacterial species *Staphylococcus aureus* and *Staphylococcus epidermis* to the surfaces of implants have been identified as the cause of approximately half of the infections associated with implants [Ball, Chapman et al.]. Bacterial adhesion is facilitated by adsorption of either human proteins or bacterial proteins on the implant surface. The protein acts as an intermediate bonding agent and in some cases, carbohydrates may also function in a similar manner [Chapman et al.]. Recent research has revealed that bacteria such as *Pseudomonas aeruginosa* (an agent of infection in contact lenses and lungs), secrete DNA as a bonding agent [Whitechurch et al. 2002]. The double helical structure of DNA presumably provides much scope for molecular entanglement, the basis of stickiness.

Polyurethane displays the rare characteristic of poor adsorption by proteins, this inhibits contamination of polyurethane by bacteria [Ball 2001, Chapman et al. 2001]. The same characteristic is shared by polyethylene glycol, which can be painted on to surfaces as a protective coating [Ball 2001, Chapman et al., 2001]. Current work on the development of coatings to suppress protein adsorption and thereby suppress bacterial infection [Chapman et al., 2001] or haemostasis [Spencer et al.], is based on the deposition of extremely thin polymer coatings. Candidate polymers are polyamine functionalized with acetyl chloride [Chapman et al.] and a co-polymer poly-lysine-g-poly (ethylene glycol) [Spencer et al.]. The polyamine coating is separated from the underlying metal surface by an intermediary self-assembled-monolayer (SAM) of mercaptohexadecanoic acid. There is still no known material, which completely prevents bacteria from absorbing on its surface [Chapman et al. 2001].

The ability of bacteria to strongly adhere to biomaterial surfaces has major implications for sterilization procedures. It is extremely difficult to completely wash off bacteria with flowing fluid unless very high shear rates can be generated in the liquid. The intense flow of liquid may also engender problems of biomaterial contamination by the fluid. Sterilization procedures involving high temperature or ionizing radiation are more effective, killing the bacteria in-situ. Residual bacterial endotoxins (toxic cellular constituents of bacterial cells) could in theory still cause problems to the patient.

3.6 Biocorrosion

The aqueous saline environment of the human body predisposes most metals to some form of corrosion. Aqueous corrosion would be further accelerated where the implant contains crevices or is located in a position where tissue fluid velocities are high, e.g. a cardiac implant. Any implant located in the stomach would have to be resistant to very low pH (high acidity). The organic components of tissue fluids, in particular the proteins, are observed to enhance corrosion beyond levels associated with non-living systems. This phenomenon is termed *biocorrosion* where a complex interaction between the inorganic and organic constitutents of tissue fluids dominates the corrosion process. Biocorrosion is undesirable not only because of the degradation of the biomaterial, but also because of the release of metal ions into the tissue fluids. Most metals are non-toxic provided that they remain in the solid state as a metal or an oxide. A common example is stainless steel cutlery, which is non-toxic despite the presence of chromium. Metal ions however show completely different levels of toxicity because of their direct interference with the metabolism.

An example of biocorrosion is commonly found in orthodontic teeth retainers that are made of stainless steel [Kusy et al., 2002]. The normally passive stainless steel was found to be partially covered by bacterial films. The bacterial films were located in mottled regions of the stainless steel, where surface analysis revealed preferential loss of chromium and nickel from the steel due to corrosion. It is believed that the coverage of the metal surface by bacterial films induced the formation of electrochemical corrosion cells that were strong enough to de-passivate the stainless steel. An electrochemical corrosion cell could be formed from an anodic region of surface covered by bacterial cells with the exposed remainder of the surface becoming cathodic.

3.7 Summary

There is a high level of interaction between most biomaterials and the host tissues, much of which is harmful to both the tissues and the organisms. The biomaterials may release toxins in the form of metal ions or organic species, but in most cases this can be controlled by the careful selection of non-toxic materials for use as biomaterials. A more pernicious problem is the colonization of biomaterials by bacteria. While the body has evolved a wide range of physical, biochemical and cellular defences against bacteria, the novel, the artificial nature of biomaterials may present an opportunity for bacteria to evade these defences. The flat surface of many implants presents a favourable site for bacteria to colonize and become extremely robust against any counter-measures by the surrounding tissues or host body. The consequences of colonization are (i) chronic or possibly acute infection of the patient and (ii) degradation of the biomaterial by processes such as biocorrosion.

References

Ian Allan, Michael Wilson, Hubert newman, "Particulate Bioglass[®] reduces the viability of bacterial biofilms formed on its surface in an *in vitro* model", Clinical Oral Implants Research, 2002, Vol. 13, No. 1, pp. 53-58.

H.C. Amstutz and P.Grigoris, Metal on metal bearings in hip arthroplasty, Clinical Orthopaedics and related research, 1996, Vol. 329S, pp. S11-S34.

S.H. Arshad, Allergy, an illustrated colour text, 2002, publ. Churchill Livingstone (Harcourt Health Sciences, Elsevier Science), Amsterdam.

P. Ball, Chemistry: non-stick hips, Nature Science Update, 28 February 2001, www.nature.com/nsu/010301/010301.html

J.R. Batchelor, Private communication, 2003.

CDC, National Center for Infection Diseases, Centers for Disease Control and Prevention, http://www.cdc.gov/ncidod/diseases/ebv.htm 27th October, 2002.

R.G. Chapman, E. Ostuni, M.N. Liang, G. Meluleni, E. Kim, L. Yan, G. Pier, H.S. Warren and G.M. Whitesides, Polymeric thin films that resist the adsorption of proteins and the adhesion of bacteria, Langmuir, 2001, Vol. 17, No. 4, pp. 1225-1233.

Mark S. Coyne, Soil Microbiology an exploratory approach, Delmar Publishers, New York, USA, 1999.

A.K. Dillow, F. Dehghani, J.S. Hrkach, N.R. Foster and R. Langer, Bacterial inactivation by using near and supercritical caron dioxide, Proc. National Academy of Sciences of the USA, 1999, Vol. 96, pp. 10344-10348.

William F. Ganong, A review of medical physiology, 19th edition, Appleton and Lange, 1999, Stamford, Connecticut, USA.

L.N. Gilbertson, Wear of polyethylene in Total Hip Replacement, Research Laboratories of Zimmer Inc., Warsaw, Indiana, 1995, http://www.zimmer.com/images/wearpoly.pdf

David Gott, Biodegradation and Toxicokinetic studies, Chapter 3, pp. 43-63 in Biocompatibility Assessment of Medical Devices and Materials, edit. Julian H. Braybrook, John Wiley and Sons, 1997, Chichester, United Kingdom.

O.A. Goeau-Brissonniere and M. Coggia, Arterial Prosthetic infections, Chapter 7, pp. 127-144, Infections associated with indwelling medical devices, 3rd edition, edit. F.A. Waldwogel and A.L. Bisno, 2000, publ. ASM Press, Washington D.C., USA.

A.W. Karchmer, Infections of prosthetic heart valves, Chapter 8, pp. 145-172, Infections associated with indwelling medical devices, 3rd edition, edit. F.A. Waldwogel and A.L. Bisno, 2000, publ. ASM Press, Washington D.C., USA.

N.-P. Huang, R. Michel, J. Voros, M. Textor, R. Hofer, A. Rossi, D.L. Elbert, J.A. Hubbell and N.D. Spencer, Poly (L-lysine) - *g* - poly (ethylene glycol) layers on metal oxide surfaces: surface-analytical characterization and resistance to serum and fibrinogen adsorption, Langmuir, 2001, Vol. 17, pp. 489-498.

Steven M. Jones, Marina Morgan, Tom J. Humphrey, Hilary Lappin-Scott, Effect of vancomycin and rifampicin on meticillin-resistant Staphylococcus aureus biofilms, The Lancet, Vol. 357, No. 9249, 6th January 2001, research letter.

G.L. Kenausis, J. Voros, D.L. Elbert, N. Huang, R. Hofer, L. Ruiz-Taylor, M. Textor, J.A. Hubbell and N.D. Spencer, Poly (L-lysine) - *g* - poly (ethylene glycol) layers on metal oxide surfaces: Attachment mechanism and effects of polymer architecture on resistance to protein adsorption, Journal of Physical Chemistry, Series B, 2000, Vol. 104, pp. 3298-3309.

R.P. Kusy, W.W. Ambrose, L.A. LaVanier, J.G. Newman and J.Q. Whitley, Analyses of rampant corrosion in stainless-steel retainers of orthodontic patients, *Journal of Biomedical Materials Research*, 2002, Vol. 62, No. 1, pp. 106-118.

Ceclia Larsson, Marco Esposito Haihong Liao and Peter Thomsen, " The Titanium-Bone Interface In-Vivo", in *Titanium in Medicaine*, Ed. D.M.Brunette, P.Tengvall, M.Textor and P.Thomsen, 2001, 588-648 Springer Publications.

J.B. Lewis, T.M. Randol, P.E. Lockwood and J.C. Wataha, Effect of subtoxic concentrations of metal ions on NFKB activation in THP-1 human monocytes, *Journal of Biomedical Materials Research*, 2002, Vol. 64A, No. 2, pp. 217-224.

E.J. Marieb, Human Anatomy and Physiology, Benjamin and Cummings Publishing Inc, 1989, California USA.

Michael McCarthy, Breaking up the bacterial happy home, The Lancet, Vol. 357, No. 9273, 23 June 2001, Feature article.

T.J. Nowak and A.G. Handford, Pathophysiology, Concepts and applications for health professionals, 2004, publ. McGraw-Hill, New York, United States of America.

Peter Parham, The immune system, Garland Publishing / Elsevier Science, New York, USA, 2000.

Pang B.K. and Freeman.S, "Oral lichenoid lesions caused by allergy to mercury in amalgam fillings", *Contact Dermitits*, 1995, Vol. 33, No. 6 pp. 423-427

Judy E. Perkin, The latex and food allergy connection, *Journal of the American Dietetic Association*, 2000, Vol. 100, No. 11, pp. 381-384.

B.D. Ratner, A.S. Hoffman, F.J. Shoen and J.E. Lemmons, ed. Biomaterials Science: An introduction to Materials in Medicine, Academic Press, 1996, pp. 415-420.

R.M. Rose, E.V. Goldfarb, E. Ellis and A.N. Crugnola, Radiation Sterilization and the Wear Rate of Polyethylene, Journal of Orthopaedic Research, 1984, Vol. 2, pp. 393-400.

J.M. Ross, Dept. Chemical and Biochemical Engineering, UMBC, description of research, web page
www.engr.umbc.edu/~itl/ENG/CHEM/FACULTY/MEMBERS/ross.html

C. Sittig, G. Hahner, A. Marti, M. Textor, N.D. Spencer and R. Hauert, The implant material, Ti6Al7Nb: surface microstructure, composition and properties, Journal of Materials Science: Materials in Engineering, 1999, Vol. 10, pp. 191-198.

C. Sittig, M. Textor, N.D. Spencer, M. Wieland, P.-H. Vallotton, Surface characterization of implant materials c.p. Ti, Ti-6-Al-7Nb and Ti-6Al-4V with different pretreatments, Journal of Materials Science: Materials in Medicine, 1999, Vol. 10, pp. 35-46.

Nicholas Spencer, ETH Zurich, Department of Materials, LSST, Functionalized Surfaces for Improved Biocompatibility of Titanium Implants, web page
www.surface.mat.ethz.ch/lsst/bio/functionalisation.html

J.M. Steckelberg and D.R. Osmon, Prosthetic joint infections, *in* F.A. Waldvogel and A.L. Bisno (editors), Infections associated with indwelling medical devices, 3rd edition, ASM Press (American Society for Microbiology), Washington, United States of America, 2000.

D.J. Stickler, G.L. Jones and A.D. Russell, Control of encrustation and blockage of Foley catheters, The Lancet, 2003, Vol. 361, No.9367.

http://www.thelancet.com/journal/vol361/iss9…/llan.361.9367.original research.25431.

F.A. Waldvogel and A.L. Bisno (editors), Infections associated with indwelling medical devices, 3rd edition, ASM Press (American Society for Microbiology), Washington, United States of America, 2000.

H.G. Wang, K.T. Wan and K.K. Liu, Osmotic swelling: a new method to characterize cell-substratum adhesion, Proc. 10th International Conference on Biomedical Engineering, Singapore, edit. JCH Goh, publ. National University of Singapore, 6-9 Dec. 2000, Singapore, pp.89-90.

Cynthia B. Whitechurch, Tim Tolker-Nielsen, Paula C. Ragas, John S. Mattick, Extracellular DNA required for bacterial film formation, Science, 2002, Vol. 295, page 1487-1489 / New Scientist News 19:00 21 February 2002, Sticky job revealed for DNA, Rachel Nowak.
http://www.newscientist.com/news/news.jsp?id=ns99991962
(Accessed 26th February 2002)

Chapter 4

Orthopaedic Prostheses

4.1 Introduction

The human skeleton consists of rigid bones that are joined by joints, which can rotate to enable movement. When these joints become unable to articulate (i.e., rotation of a synovial joint) because of disease or injury, human movement becomes difficult or even impossible. The experience of pain when flexing joints, swelling and deformity in joints is known as arthritis. Arthritis is a major contributor to healthcare costs because very few people are directly killed by arthritis, instead they lose in varying degrees the ability to care for themselves. The restoration of free and painless human movement by the implantation of artificial joints has become a very important application of biomaterials. Some joints, such as the hip and knee have proven amenable to the implantation of prostheses, while other joints such as between spinal vertebrae remain problematic. As discussed in Chapter 1, orthopaedic prostheses should offer a functional life of at least 20 years to match the life span of most patients. This presents a considerable problem for most biomedical materials. Part of the difficulty in formulating a suitable biomaterial arises from the lack of understanding of the service conditions of orthopaedic implants. In this chapter, a comparison of natural and artificial joints is presented together with current understanding of the long-term service problems of orthopaedic biomaterials.

4.2　Synovial lubrication and origins of arthritis

4.2.1　*Structure of a synovial joint*

Synovial lubrication occurs inside synovial joints, which are found inside the ankle, the knee, the hip, the shoulder, and any other moving joint such as in the fingers. The common features of all synovial joints are; A synovial capsule which separates the synovial joint from adjacent tissues, layers of cartilage at the end of each bone and synovial fluid which fills the space between the cartilage and the synovial capsule. The synovial joint is shown schematically in Figure 4.1.

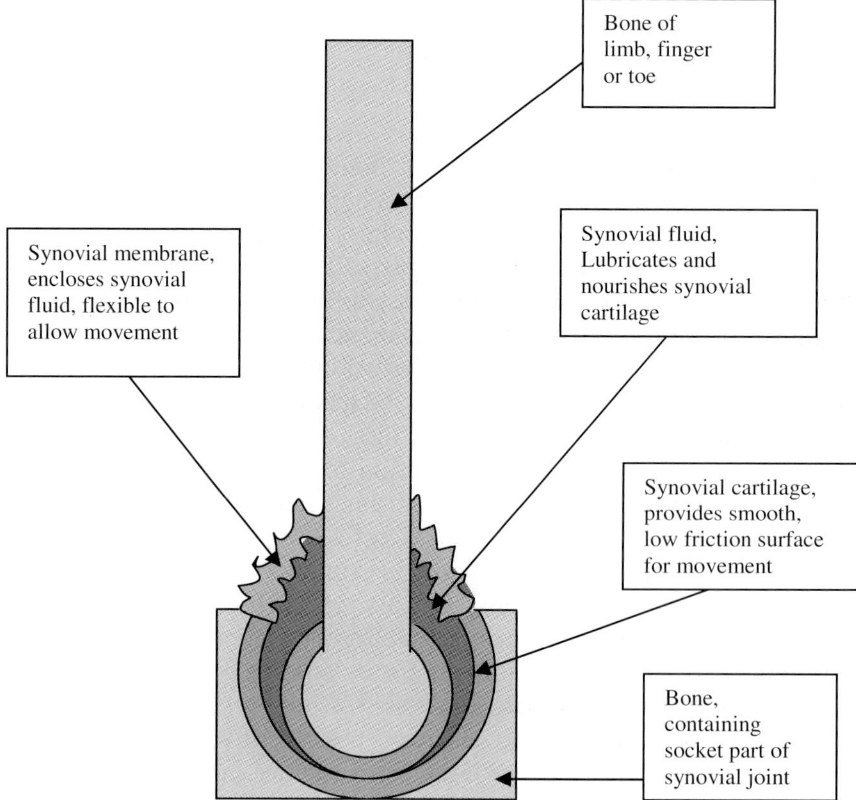

Fig 4.1.　Schematic illustration of a synovial joint.

The synovial joint is avascular, i.e. lacks a network of capillaries to convey blood, but is instead nourished by a flow of synovial fluid and diffusion of nutrients through the cartilage. Synovial fluid is related to blood serum but differs fundamentally in cellular and protein content. The cellular content of synovial fluid is normally much lower than for serum, synovial fluid cellular content is only high for arthritic patients, especially rheumatoid arthritis. The clotting system of serum based on fibrin is largely absent in synovial fluid where albumin is the most common protein. Synovial fluid is also rich in hyaluronic acid and some proteoglycans, which render the fluid highly viscous with a strong visco-elastic characteristic. Proteoglycans are a complex form of polysaccharide. It appears that synovial fluid has evolved to contain components, which contribute to lubrication with the minimum of damage by the intense shearing involved. Entities, which are vulnerable to shearing damage, such as cells are largely excluded from synovial fluid. There is however almost certainly some degradation of synovial fluid contents by shearing and a function of the synovial capsule may be to prevent escape into the external tissue of substances modified by shearing.

The cartilage has a much larger proportion of extra-cellular matrix than most other human tissues. The synovial joint resembles a passive structure, which performs a mechanical function, as opposed to an active site of biochemical activity, like most human organs. Despite the relative passivity, there is significant metabolic and cellular activity in the synovial joint, which has a direct effect on synovial lubrication and durability of the synovial joint.

4.2.1.1 Synovial lubrication

Efficient natural lubrication has long been recognized as a basic requirement for the unrestricted movement of synovial joints [Mow, 1969 and Dumbleton 1981]. Synovial lubrication enables human joints to articulate with coefficients of friction as low as 0.001 over a service lifetime of several decades. This is a superior performance to most manufactured bearings. The low friction coefficient and durability of synovial lubrication cannot be attributed to one substance alone, e.g. the synovial fluid, but is instead a system characteristic. Studies on sheep cartilage [Kirk and Stachowiak, 1994] has revealed that cartilage by itself has extremely poor sliding properties and wears very rapidly when lubrication fails. Earlier works revealed that synovial fluid is poor at lubricating artificial materials, but it was later found that synovial fluid is an effective lubricant of cartilage [Stachowiak, et.al., 1994]. Model studies of synovial protein solutions lubricating conventional polymer biomaterials have demonstrated that proteins are associated with elevated friction coefficients and degrade under sliding to cause corrosive wear of the polymers [Chandrasekaran and Batchelor, 2002]. The system characteristic of remarkably low friction therefore remains poorly understood. It is believed that the synovial lubrication is based on hydrodynamic lubrication where the high viscosity of human synovial fluid compared to water is significant [Dowson, Unsworth and Wright, 1975]. Hydrodynamic lubrication is a physical phenomenon where a large pressure is generated when fluid is dragged by viscous forces into the enclosed space between two sliding surfaces (for a full discussion of hydrodynamic lubrication refer to, Stachowiak and Batchelor 2000). However, synovial fluid is not a simple Newtonian fluid but contains numerous proteins such as albumin and the globulins, which react to viscous shearing and alter the rheology of the synovial fluid. A Newtonian fluid is one, which displays a linear proportionality between shear rate and viscous shear stress. The theory of hydrodynamic lubrication is modeled on Newtonian fluids. It is believed that the intense shearing, which occurs in the synovial liquid trapped between the sliding cartilage surfaces, causes the molecules of albumin and other proteins to uncoil and form a network of tangled molecules [O'Neill and Stachowiak 1996, O'Neill et al. 1989]. This process is likened to the stiffening of egg white after vigorous whisking and causes the synovial fluid to form a mechanically robust film that is capable of separating the cartilage surfaces.

A form of hydrodynamic lubrication, which may be unique to synovial joints, is the so-called 'weeping mechanism' of lubrication [McCutchen 1959]. The physical structure of synovial cartilage can be likened to a sponge [Maroudas, 1976] where the liquid is held within a porous matrix by ionic forces. Under heavy loads, the liquid is driven out of the cartilage to lubricate the synovial joint.

While hydrodynamic lubrication and its variants involve a fluid or semi-fluid film that is at least one micrometer thick, other lubrication mechanisms are significant when the opposing cartilage surfaces make very close contact. Such close contact might occur under extreme loads or when the viscosity of the synovial fluid is reduced (e.g. by illness). Synovial proteins may adsorb on the cartilage surface to form a semi-solid film, which will also affect the friction coefficient. There is experimental evidence that one or more glycoproteins enhance the lubricating effect of synovial fluid [Swann, Hendren et al. 1981]. Hyaluronic acid, which is a major component of synovial fluid, is also believed to act in a comparable manner to the proteins [Swann, Radin et al. 1974].

The synovial fluid is not the only source of molecular species to form adsorbed layers, instead some of the material may originate from within the cartilage. The surface of the articular cartilage is covered with a thin phospholipid layer and below this layer there are discrete vesicles (particles) of phospho-lipid within the cartilage matrix [Kirk, Wilson and Stachowiak, 1993]. The surface phospholipid layer consists of numerous spheroidal particles packed together to form a continuous lamina in healthy synovial joints [Ballantine and Stachowiak, 2002]. These phospho-lipids are found to reduce the sliding friction of synovial cartilage in the absence of significant lubrication by the synovial fluid [Hills and Butler 1984, Williams, Powell and LaBerge 1993]. Deliberate removal of the phospho-lipid layer by washing with a solvent induces rapid wear of the underlying cartilage in the absence of synovial fluid [Ballantine and Stachowiak, 2002]. In this experimental work, the synovial fluid was first removed by syringe and then the synovial cartilage was washed with an ethanol solvent. These recent findings confirm earlier experiments where greatly elevated friction was found when the articular cartilage was washed with a lipid solvent [Little et al., 1969].

As can be seen, there are several competing mechanisms of lubrication within the synovial joint. The most significant of these mechanisms are illustrated schematically in Figure 4.2. It may also be evident that it is very difficult to produce an artificial synovial implant that functions in a similar manner to the natural synovial joint.

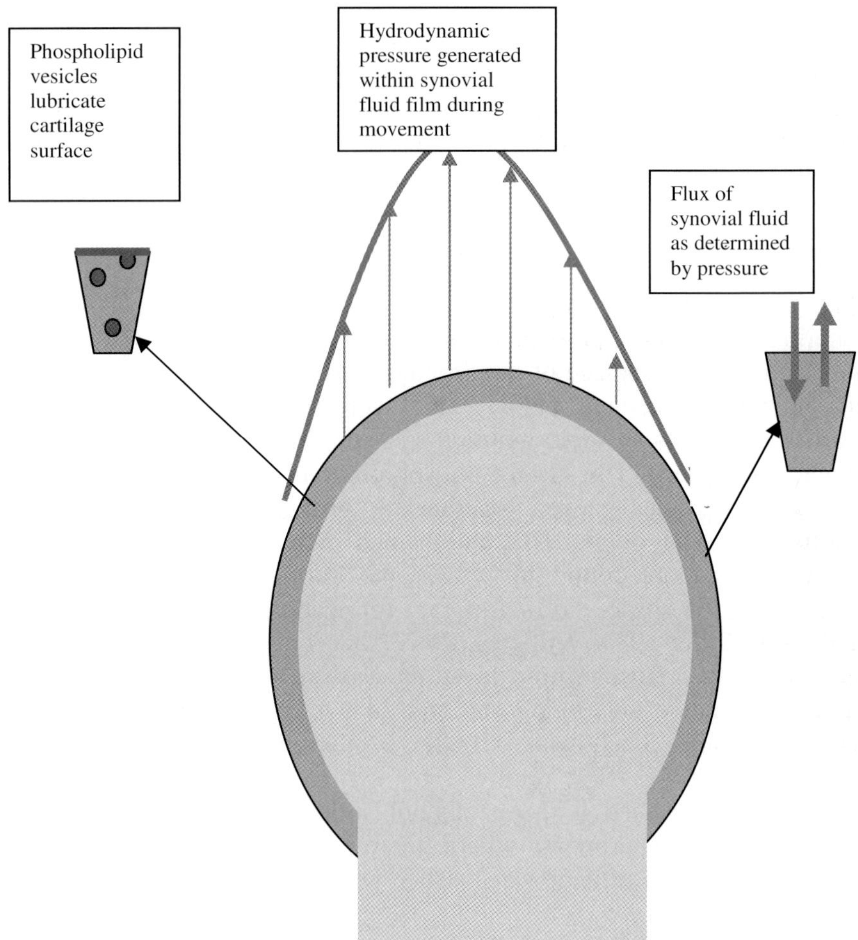

Fig 4.2. Mechanisms of synovial lubrication.

4.2.1.2   Causes of arthritis

The causes of arthritis, its aetiology, are complex and still not fully understood. It is known that there are two basic and distinct causes of arthritis, inflammation and mechanical damage [Batchelor and Stachowiak 1996]. Inflammation is associated with rheumatoid arthritis and involves auto-immunity where the immune system of the body is induced to attack a synovial joint instead of microbes and viruses as it is supposed to do. Rheumatoid arthritis causes the synovial capsule to become permeable and allow cells from adjacent tissue and circulation systems to invade the synovial joint. The cellular content of the synovial fluid then rises precipitately with many of the cells involved in tissue inflammation. These cells then proceed to attack the cartilage, which is also stressed by the loss of lubrication from the weakened synovial fluid. Mechanical damage is associated with osteo-arthritis where either trauma (a limb fracture) or prolonged mechanical overload initiates degradation of the articular cartilage. The released cartilage particles induce a change in the cellular content and enzymatic of the synovial fluid, which is a response to try and destroy the cartilage particles by extra metabolic activity. The same processes, which destroy suspended cartilage particles, also damage the bulk cartilage and initiate arthritis [Otterness et al. 2000, Evans 1991, Maiotti et al. 2000]. The causes of the sensitivity of synovial fluid to suspended cartilage particles remain unknown, this sensitivity makes synovial fluid different from an artificial lubricant which passively accepts wear particles. It has been suggested that suspended particles would impede network formation by proteins under shearing and so reduce the effective viscosity of the synovial fluid [Stachowiak, 1995].   Some mechanical loading is essential for healthy function of the synovial joints, it appears that only extremes of mechanical load cause destruction of the cartilage. Impulsive (impact) loads such as caused by jumping from great heights are known to initiate 'budding' of cartilage where particles are released from cartilage, which has sustained subsurface damage.   The damage processes of rheumatoid arthritis and osteo-arthritis are illustrated schematically in Figure 4.3.

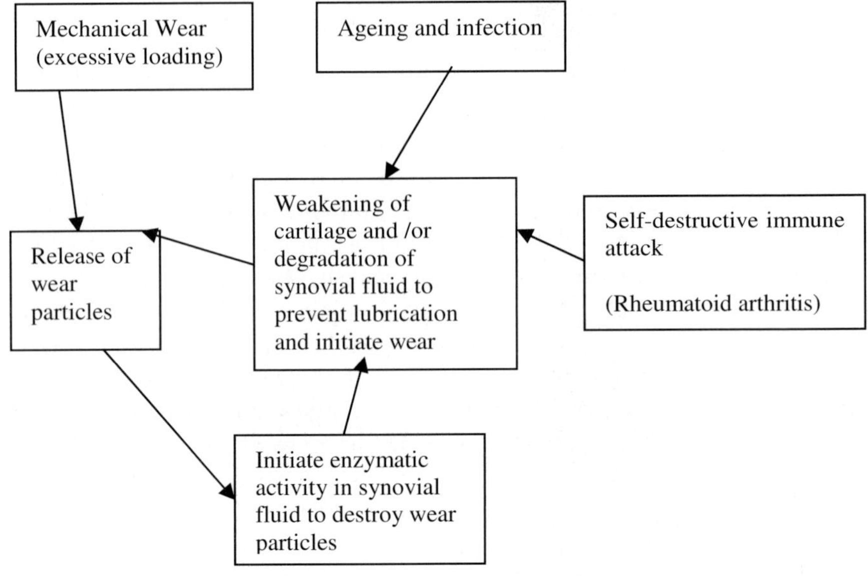

Fig 4.3. Causes and damage processes of arthritis.

4.3 Materials for orthopaedic prostheses

Orthopaedic endoprostheses, e.g. the 'artificial hip', are generally designed as a socket or cup and a ball, which is also fitted with a stem to be inserted in the bone. Illustrations of hip implants and knee implants are provided in Figure 4.4.

This design has a substantial influence on the selection of materials for the prostheses. While the cup sustains mostly compressive stresses, the ball and the stem, in particular, have to sustain tensile stresses from bending and rapidly varying or impulsive loads. The socket and stem must therefore be made of a material with high strength under mechanical fatigue and good toughness. These requirements virtually determine the use of strong metals for the stem as opposed to any other materials, although it is possible to fit a threaded socket of a non-metal to the stem. The mechanical loads on prosthesis for the hip are shown schematically in Figure 4.5.

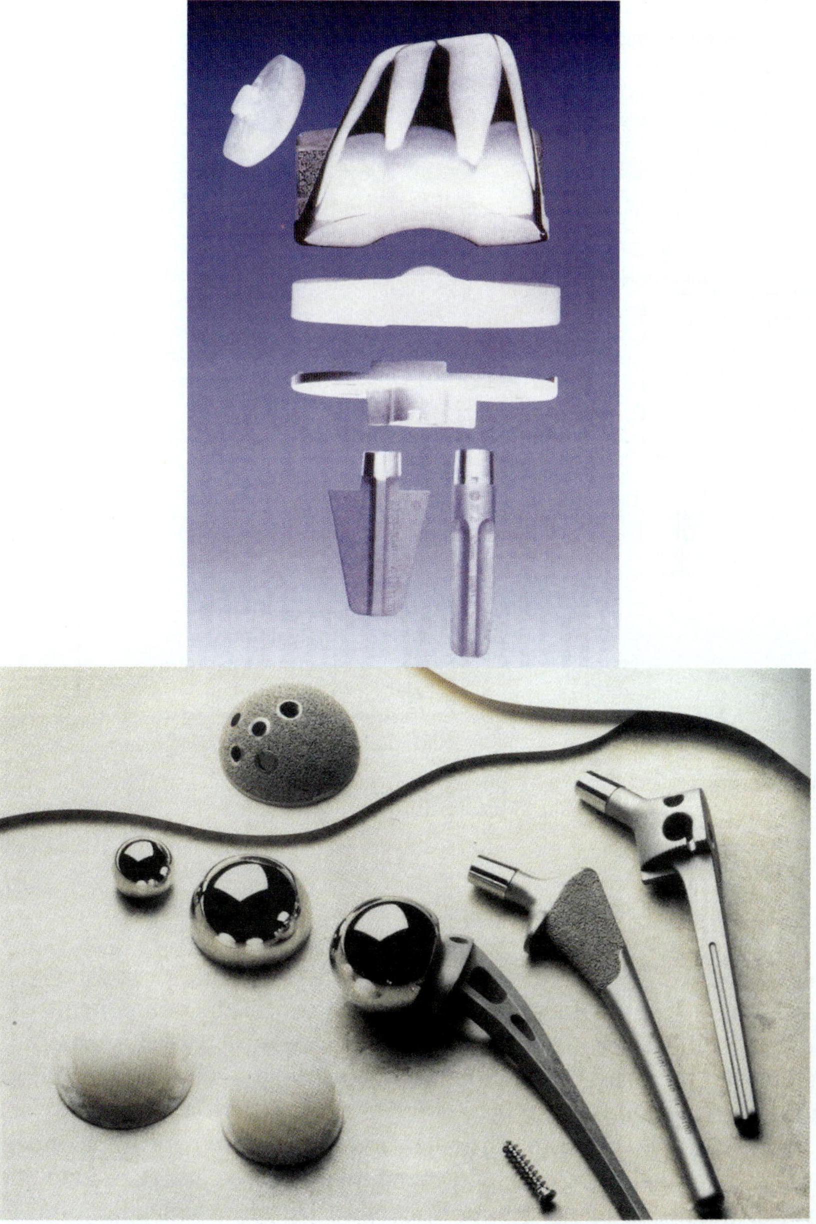

Fig 4.4. Orthopaedic implants for the knee (upper picture) and the hip (lower picture). By courtesy of Dr Stephen Hsu, National Institute of Standards and Technology, USA.

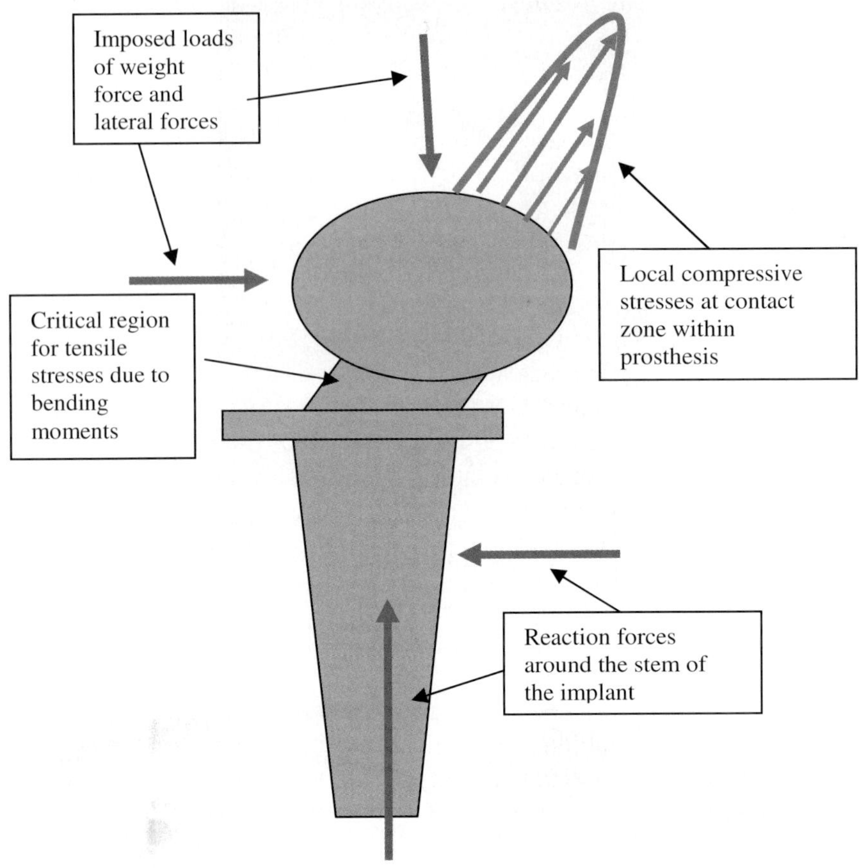

Fig 4.5. Design and mechanical loads on the 'artificial hip'.

A minimum level of toughness is required for all the components of the prosthesis, aluminium oxide (alumina) has been tested as a material for the cup but there are doubts whether its brittleness would cause chipping and cup fracture during service [Morita et al. 2003]. The complex shape of the socket and stem in particular and the requirement of accuracy of form and good surface finish on the spherical surfaces necessitate a high level of quality in manufacture. Since the size of orthopaedic joints vary between individuals, the mass production of prostheses faces considerable difficulty.

4.3.1 *Implant materials chosen to optimize synovial lubrication*

There are a wide variety of materials in use for orthopaedic prostheses, most materials used are chosen on the basis of high hardness and wear resistance but there are other types of materials used as well. In one innovative attempt to enhance hydrodynamic lubrication inside an orthopaedic prosthesis, a material with low elastic modulus but high strength is slid against a counterface with a high elastic modulus [Unsworth et al.1987, Blamey et al. 1991]. The large difference in mechanical rigidity causes the surface of the softer material to become almost perfectly aligned with the harder material. Hydrodynamic lubrication is enhanced on rotating systems when the opposing surfaces are closely conformal and there are no sharp projections from either surface. When the opposing surfaces are closely conformal, the maximum value of contact pressure is reduced and the hydrodynamic pressure field extends over most of the sliding interface instead of being concentrated around the load line. Hydrodynamic lubrication is usually limited by maximum contact pressure, when this pressure is exceeded there is a collapse of the hydrodynamic film and high friction results. Unsworth's model of hydrodynamic lubrication for an orthopaedic prosthesis is illustrated in Figure 4.6.

It is found that a combination of a polyurethane cup and a metal ball gives a low friction coefficient and low wear under loads and speeds typical of a hip joint while the joint is moving. Unacceptable levels of wear and friction occur at the initial moments of movement when hydrodynamic lubrication is ineffective [Unsworth 1998]. Hydrodynamic lubrication requires a minimum speed to be functional. Polyurethane has very poor wear resistance in sliding contact and would need to be covered with a low friction coating. At present it appears that there is no suitable coating for polyurethane, which has greatly limited its use as an implant material.

4.3.2 *Wear-resistant materials for orthopaedic implants*

Whereas Unsworth and co-workers have tried to develop a materials system, which is matched to the characteristics of synovial fluid, most other orthopaedic biomaterials have been developed to function without support from the synovial fluid. The main types of materials used are metal on polymer, metal on metal and ceramics.

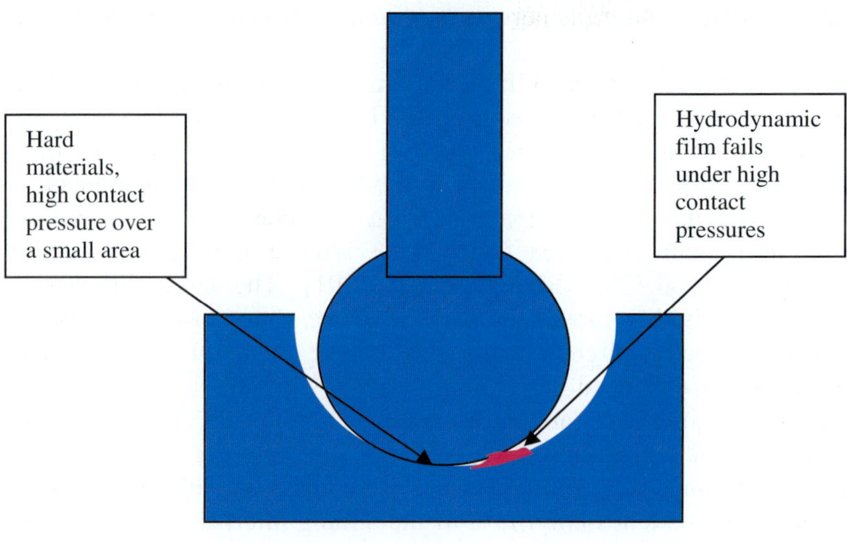

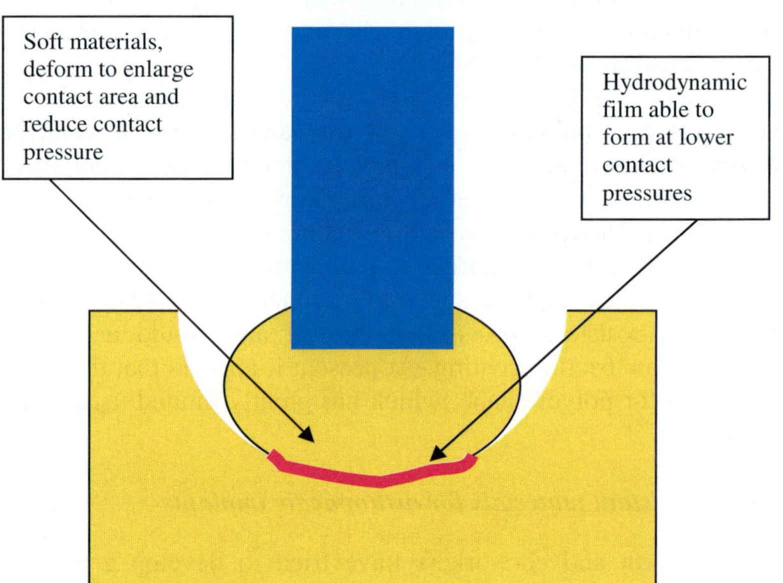

Fig 4.6. Enhancement of hydrodynamic lubrication in an orthopaedic prosthesis.

4.3.2.1 <u>Metals and polymers</u>

A popular materials combination for the hip prosthesis and knee prosthesis is a metal socket sliding against a cup of Ultra-High Molecular Weight Polyethylene (UHMWPE). UHMWPE is a polymer with a molecular weight exceeding 1 million units (*Daltons*) and is used as wear resistant material for bearings. UHMWPE is also tough and strong compared to other polymers, it is highly resistant to corrosion at ambient temperatures. Metals used to construct the stem and socket comprise of cobalt, vanadium and titanium alloys. A common Cobalt alloy includes Chromium and Molybdenum in the alloy. An alloy formulation used by at least one manufacturer of implants consists of 28% Molybdenum, 6% Chromium in Cobalt [Savarini et al., 2003]. These metals are chosen for their high strength and corrosion resistance and comparative lack of toxicity. The lesser volume of wear debris from metal-on-metal hips as opposed to metal-on-polymer hips renders them suitable for younger more active patients. However, there is concern at the release of metal ions such as chromium and cobalt into the patient [Savarini et al., 2003]. It is fortunate that the toxic element aluminum, which is also present in the alloy, was not released in significant quantities [Savarini et al., 2003]. The cost of metals, such as cobalt, is high but is of less economic significance than the costs of precision manufacture and of surgical placement of the prosthesis, not to mention revision (surgical replacement) of the prosthesis.

4.3.2.2 <u>Ceramic materials</u>

Engineering ceramics such as alumina, zirconia-toughened alumina are used as screw-on sockets for metal stems or as cups. Pure zirconia is unsuitable and it must be alloyed with other ceramics to achieve sufficient strength. Y-TZP or Yttria-toughened-zirconia-polycrystal is widely used for this purpose. The benefits of using alumina include its high chemical stability and lack of toxicity. The combination of ceramic sliding material is important for the control of wear and friction. It is found that zirconium dioxide (zirconia) generates high wear and friction when sliding against itself and a more suitable combination is zirconia sliding against alumina [Morita et al. 2003]. Alumina sliding against alumina is acceptable because the surface of the alumina reacts with water and forms soft, lubricious aluminium hydroxides [Gates et al.

1989]. Alumina matrix composites have also been introduced where zirconium dioxide is blended into an alumina matrix [Stewart et al., 2003].

4.3.2.3 Composite materials

The high density and elastic modulus of cobalt, vanadium and titanium alloys when compared to bone, has led researchers to consider substitute materials, which closely resembles bone. The large difference in material properties between prosthesis and bone causes problems of bone resorption, which are discussed below. Carbon fibre composites have been proposed for the stem of the prosthesis [Ramakrishnan et al. 2003]. The elastic modulus and density of the stem can be adjusted by varying the density and weaving of the carbon fibres in the composite.

4.3.2.4 Cementation of implants and bioactive coatings

The implants can be classified into two categories namely cemented implant and cementless implant. The stem of the prosthesis requires bonding to the surrounding bone and traditionally poly-methacrylate cement is used for this purpose. This type of implant falls under the classification of cemented implants. The cement often does not function well and release particles of polymethacrylate into the surrounding tissue, which often becomes inflamed as a result. Another typical problem associated with cemented implants is the progressive loosening of the implant upon release of particles from the cement and wear of the implant leading to catastrophic failure of implant. Metals do not bond well with bone and other tissues, metal implants are typically surrounded by a thin, quiescent, or possibly necrotic layer that acts as a buffer between the metal and living tissue [Williams, 1987]. If a metal is coated with a *bio-active* material, where bio-activity denotes the tendency of tissue to grow merge with the material, then it is possible for the coated metal to bond strongly to the tissue. A bioactive material can be either osteo inductive or osteo conductive and promote tissue bonding and growth. Bio-active materials were first developed by Hench and co-workers after Hench observed that silica exo-skeletons of marine organisms formed on templates consisting of amino acids. For the human body, bio-active materials are a range of glasses containing varying compositions of silicon dioxide, phosphate, calcium oxide and sodium oxide. Bio-active materials are further classified into materials which enhance bone growth around them, and materials which merely allow bone to come into close contact and develop a bond. The former phenomenon is termed osteo-production and the latter is termed osteo-conduction [Hench 2001]. Osteo-conductive materials bond more slowly than osteo-producers and do not bond with connective tissues. It is important to attain the correct level of bio-activity for any given application since an excessively bio-active material is likely to become resorbed by the body.

4.3.2.5   <u>Bioactive coatings from hydroxyapatite and related materials</u>

A bio-active material that has attracted considerable interest is hydroxyapatite, which is a form of calcium phosphate. Calcium phosphate, i.e., hydroxyapatite, is a major constituent of bone, a metal implant that is coated with hydroxyapatite and placed inside bone does show rapid growth of bone cells into the hydroxyapatite coating. Once the growth of the bone cells is complete, the coated metal becomes very strongly bonded to bone. The coated apatite may eventually be resorbed by the body, which would in the long-term leave bare metal in contact with the bone [Savarini, Fini et al., 2003]. Hydroxyapatite is non-toxic but advanced coating techniques are required to bond a strongly adhering coating to a metal. Plasma spraying appears to be the most effective technique, depositing hydroxyapatite as a porous coating well suited to the ingress of bone cells [Kweh et.al, 2000]. It should be noted however that high temperature decomposition during plasma spraying impede the deposition of hydroxyapatite coatings and other deposition processes such as electrostatic spray deposition may be more suitable [Leeuwenburgh et al., 2003]. Excessive roughness of the coated apatite inhibits bone regrowth while particles of coating may become detached and inhibit bone regrowth [Savarini, Fini et al., 2003]. After regrowth of the bone around the implant, bone-to-implant bond strengths of the order of 10 MPa in shear and somewhat less than this in tension are reported [Milthorpe, 2000]. This is less than the maximum tensile strength of cortical bone, but comparable to the tensile strength of cancellous bone [Milthorpe, 2000]. Pull-out is a more likely mode of failure for a bone implant than bone fracture, even with a bio-active coating. Pull-out may not necessarily occur at the interface between bone and coating but instead between the metal and the hydroxyapatite coating. The brittleness of hydroxyapatite and its poor adhesion to metal compromise its performance as a coating [Redepenning et al., 2003].

Bio-active coatings based on hydroxyapatite have poor friction and wear properties [Fu et al., 1999.], so these coatings should not be exposed to sliding movement. Sliding movements include microscopic motion (fretting) that typically occurs between tightly fitting surfaces.

Pure hydroxyapatite coatings are now being substituted by chitosan/hydroxyapatite composites [Redepenning et al., 2003] to improve bone adhesion or by fluorohydroxyapatite coatings to improve bone integration [Savarini, Fini et al., 2003]. Finally, bioactive coatings of hydroxyapatite are not only used for orthopaedic implants but also as a component of temporary porous structures called 'scaffolds' (discussed in later chapters) for bone restoration [Maquet et al., 2003].

4.3.3 *Sterilisation of orthopaedic prostheses*

A very high degree of sterility is required for any surgical placement of orthopaedic prostheses, since any infection inside a bone will have severe consequences for a patient. Immersion in pressurized steam at approximately 120 degrees Celsius in an autoclave, fumigation by the highly toxic ethylene oxide and exposure to nuclear radiation are commonly used to sterilize biomedical materials. Irradiation by gamma rays from a Cobalt 60 source has become an accepted standard procedure for the sterilization of UHMWPE orthopaedic prostheses, since the process is efficient and does not leave any toxic residues. While gamma rays are not destructive to metals, they are known to cause embrittlement of UHMWPE via radiation-induced oxidation of the polymer molecules [Pascaud et al. 1997]. It has been concluded that the level of radiation used in sterilization is not sufficient to cause a significant increase in oxidative degradation of UHMWPE in service. UHMWPE is found to oxidize significantly over service periods of 15 years or more even without significant initial oxidation [Oonishi et al. 2001]. Wear resistance does however appear to be significantly degraded by gamma-ray sterilization with a 5-fold increase in wear rate for UHMWPE pins in uni-directional sliding [Besong et al. 1998]. This data is based on in-vitro laboratory tests, it is difficult to say whether a comparable increase in wear rate would be found for real prostheses after service in-vivo. In-vivo comparisons of the effect of sterilization would be difficult because of the risk of infections to patients.

4.3.3.1   Highly cross–linked UHMWPE and enhanced wear resistance

The utility of gamma-radiation extends beyond sterilization to conversely, enhancing the wear resistance. The critical step appears to be combine gamma irradiation with subsequent remelting and / or surface melting with an electron beam to induce a high level of cross-linking between the polyethylene molecules [Muratoglu et al., 2001; Hastings et al., 1999, Di Maio et al., 1998]. The level of radiation used for cross linking is typically 100 kGy, which is significantly greater than the 30 kGy radiation dose used for sterilization [Kurtz et al, 1999; Villarraga et al., 2003]. Currently, greatly enhanced wear resistance is claimed for hip prostheses but there is limited understanding of how the treatment process increases the wear resistance. The bulk material properties of the cross-linked UHMWPE also differs from the untreated UHMWPE with a less plastic deformation before failure under low cycle fatigue (less than 10,000 cycles) [Villarraga et al., 2003].

4.4   Fracture of orthopaedic prostheses

Orthopaedic prostheses must withstand highly variable loads, just like the original joints. High fatigue strength of orthopaedic prosthesis is critical for active users, who participate in physical activities involving jumping. Fortunately, it appears that the metal alloys used for orthopaedic prostheses have sufficiently high fatigue strength for the prosthesis to survive a very long period of service. Post-operative monitoring of patients who have received knee prostheses, indicate that the primary causes of failure are prosthesis wear and deep infection of the tissues adjacent to the implanted prosthesis [Van Loon et al., 2000]. The knee prosthesis did not possess a stem however, and it is possible that prosthesis with stems that are subject to bending would be more vulnerable to fracture. Early fatigue fracture of femoral stems has been reported with CoCr forged stem. The failure is mainly concentrated at the neck of the stem. The failure is mainly attributed to high residual stresses accumulated during manufacture [Lee and Kim, 2001]. Cast cobalt-chromium alloys have also been observed to be prone to fatigue fracture, especially where microstructural imperfections generate stress concentrations [Swarts et al., 2001].

Orthopaedic prosthesis fracture appears to be mostly found in finger prostheses. The most commonly used prosthesis for arthritic fingers is the Swanson prosthesis, which consists of a flexible length of silicone elastomer that bends to allow finger movement [Swanson, 1972]. Repeated flexure of the elastomer causes its eventual fracture. The maximum reported incidence of fracture in Swanson prostheses is 82% after five years [Kay et al., 1978]. In an effort to prevent this fracture, a replacement for the Swanson prosthesis involving articulating joints is being developed [Joyce et al., 2002].

4.5   Wear and corrosion of orthopaedic prostheses

In most instances, it appears that wear is the prime cause of operational problems with orthopaedic prostheses such as the hip and knee joint. The lesser-loaded finger prosthesis is found to wear very little if at all [Joyce et al. 2002]. Corrosion is considered to be less of a problem, largely because of the deliberate choice of non-ferrous self-passivating metals for implants, such as titanium or chromium. However some evidence of corrosion in worn implants has been found. A study of new and retrieved hip prostheses revealed that corrosion-originated pits had formed on the worn surface of the implants [Koerten et al. 2002]. The cause of this is believed to be a galvanic cell formed between the implant alloy, which contained cobalt, chromium and molybdenum, and impurities containing titanium and aluminium. These impurities may have been deposited on the surface during the manufacturing process [Koerten et al. 2002]. The significance of this corrosion is the subsequent release of toxic cobalt, chromium and molybdenum into the human tissues. When a femoral implant is made of cobalt alloy, corrosion is estimated to cause a reduction in linear dimension of 100 nanometres per year [Black, 1996]. Any cobalt wear particles are also corroded to form soluble products that can have adverse effects on the body [Amstutz et al., 1996].

4.5.1   *Wear mechanisms in orthopaedic prostheses*

The significance of wear as problem of orthopaedic prostheses has been recognized ever since the pioneering work of Sir John Charnley. Charnley chose Polytetrafluoroethylene (PTFE) as the material for the cups of his hip prosthesis design since PTFE was known to have very low friction and would not release metallic wear debris unlike earlier designs using metal. Unfortunately it was not realized that PTFE also displays a very high wear rate, amongst the highest for polymers in sliding wear. PTFE is also very soft and easily suffers permanent plastic deformation. As a result of the poor characteristics of PTFE, Charnley's initial version of hip prosthesis suffered from very rapid wear and escape of large amounts of wear particles into the surrounding tissue. The excessive release of wear particles was associated with intense inflammation of the surrounding tissue and illness in the users. The hard metal socket also caused the soft PTFE lining inside the cup to be extruded to the outside. Charnley recalled hundreds of his hip prostheses and substituted UHMWPE for the PTFE [Charnley, 1961 and 1963].

Most workers have observed that synovial fluid does not provide effective lubrication for artificial materials; this results in much higher friction coefficients orthopaedic prostheses than for natural synovial joints. Model tests of UHMWPE sliding against a martensitic stainless steel have shown that the addition of synovial proteins such as albumen (used as a substitute for albumin in an experimental model of synovial fluid), gamma and alpha globulin raise the friction coefficient from the value for pure water [Batchelor and Chandrasekaran 2002.]. A high friction coefficient is associated with a high wear rate and there may be an excessively high level of frictional heat dissipation. It is possible that during heavy exercise, the temperature of the implant may be sufficiently elevated to cause thermal degradation of adjacent tissues and body fluids. A temperature rise of approximately 10 degrees Celsius is sufficient; this is negligible when compared to the frictional temperature rises occurring in sliding contact. In this context, it should be noted that the main mode of heat transfer within the human body is convection by the circulation of blood. The thermal conductivity of human tissues is low and a virtually avascular environment such as in and around an orthopaedic prosthesis would be expected to suffer from inefficient dissipation of heat. The typical values of the thermal conductivity of the bone are close to the cement at 0.3-0.6 J/m.s.K as opposed to 19 J/m.s.K for the prostheses. These values of thermal conductivity are based on artificial tissue substitutes [Craciunescu et. al., 1999; Shalek and Chien]. When heat cannot escape easily, the temperature rises until thermal conduction and possibly thermal radiation become effective. A temperature rise from room temperature (approximately 25 degrees Celsius) to body temperature of 37 degrees Celsius was found to be associated with a doubling of the wear of UHMWPE sliding against a metal counterface and lubricated by serum [Imado et al., 2000].

As discussed in Chapter 2, the human body presents a highly corrosive environment to which orthopaedic prostheses are not an exempt. A major cause of wear in the UHMWPE-metal prosthesis is aqueous corrosion of the metal which then forms oxides. It was observed in the earlier literature that these metal oxides are sufficiently hard to gouge the UHMWPE when oxide particles detach from the worn metal surface. The same oxide particles may also become embedded in the UHMWPE and then gouge the original metal surface. The roughening of the metal surface by gouging causes rapid wear of the UHMWPE [Buchanan et al, 1987; Mazzucco and Spector, 2003]. This corrosive mechanism of prosthesis wear is shown schematically in Figure 4.7.

Synovial proteins sustain physical and chemical changes under the intense shearing and heating that occurs in sliding contact between artificial materials. Tests of UHMWPE sliding against martensitic stainless steel reveal that aqueous solution of albumen and gamma globulin form lumps, which are sufficiently hard to gouge and severely wear UHMWPE [Batchelor and Chandrasekaran 2002]. There is still no precise model of lubrication within an orthopaedic prosthesis, but the overall picture appears to be of adverse interaction between synovial fluid and current prosthesis materials.

Released wear particles do not necessarily stay close to the site of wear, which is the orthopaedic implant. The larger wear particles tend to remain close to the implant while the smaller particles migrate to other tissues more distant from the implant. It is believed that these smaller particles are a cause of aseptic implant loosening and osteolysis (destruction of bone) through the initiation of tissue inflammation (discussed below) [Mabrey et al., 2001].

Tissue inflammation remains a major problem for orthopaedic implants and other types of metal implants. Recent work has found that polymers with hydrophilic surfaces engender a milder immune response by cellular macrophages than hydrophobic surfaces [Brodbeck et al.]. It is found that smaller numbers of macrophages adhere to hydrophilic surfaces than to hydrophobic surfaces. Hydrophobic surfaces repel water, which forms large droplets on the surface whereas hydrophilic surfaces attract water, which then wets the surface. A candidate hydrophilic polymer is polyacrylamide.

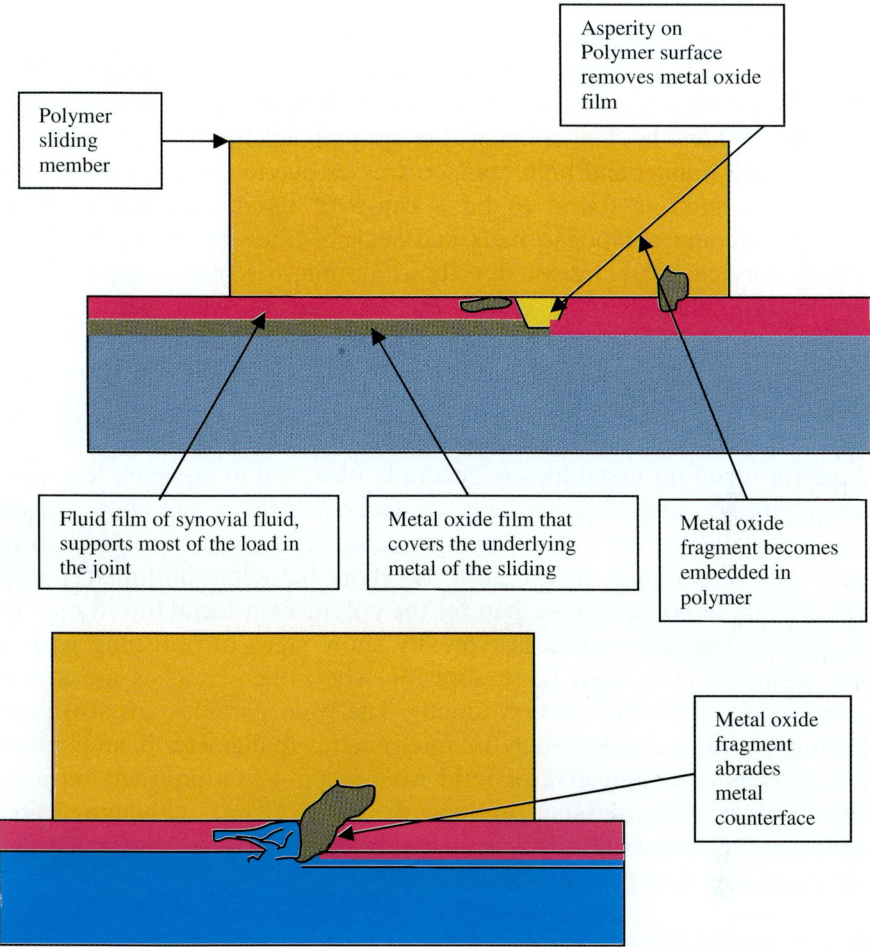

Fig 4.7.   Corrosive wear mechanism in orthopaedic prosthesis with the UHMWPE - metal sliding combination.

Wear is not only generated by tangential sliding movement between the ball and the socket but is also accentuated by separation and impact between the ball and socket. A phenomenon known as micro-separation occurs in the unloaded part of the swing cycle of the legs during walking. When the leg is swinging unloaded, any slackness in the tendons and other connective tissue may allow the ball and cup to momentarily separate. When the leg contacts the ground again, the ball and cup contact with impact and high contact stresses due to misaligned contact. Micro-separation is found to be a cause of rapid localized wear in alumina-zirconia composite balls and sockets [Stewart et al., 2003]. A critical service characteristic for these alumina-zirconia composites is the intergranular strength within the material as wear particles are mostly generated by intergranular fracture under the test conditions [Stewart et al., 2003]. The phenomenon of micro-separation is illustrated schematically in Figure 4.8.

Wear for metal-on-metal hips is generally observed to be much less than for polymer-on-metal hip implants, provided that the cobalt alloy is used and not stainless steel. The average volumetric wear of cobalt alloy metal on metal hips is measured to be about 0.3 cubic millimeters/year which is about 60 times less than for the polymer-on-metal hip [Sieber et al., 1999]. The worn surfaces typically show signs of polishing with a few scratches from third body abrasion where the scratches are a few micrometres in width (i.e. very small). The wear particles are also very small, typically being less than 0.2 micrometres in diameter [Campbell et al., 2002], this is indicative of mild wear leading to a polished surface. The friction characteristic appears to be moderate although some instances of 'squeaking hips', presumably due to stick-slip between the metal surfaces have been reported [Sieber et al., 1999].

Wear is not confined solely to the sliding interface of ball and socket, but also occurs often around the cemented stem. Ideally, the stem should be rigidly bonded to the bone by the cement but in practice the poor adhesion of PMMA cement and the presence of cracks and voids permits micro-movements. These micro-movements, which may only be on the scale of a few micrometres, are termed fretting. Fretting wear of the cement generates PMMA particles that eventually escape into the synovial joint space.

4.6 Bone substitutes

There are a number of materials referred to as bone substitutes, which are used to fill holes in bones or reinforce weak bones in a patient. Before describing these in detail however, it should be noted that bone is a complex living tissue that still cannot be fully replicated by an artificial material.

Recent research is directed to creating materials that are closely analogous to bone. Bone is modeled as a network of bone cells, osteoblasts, which have an extensive extracellular matrix of collagen that provides a base for hydroxyapatite crystals to adhere. The hydroxyapatite crystals confer hardness and strength to the bone. Collagen, which is a protein, forms long linear, or gently spiralling molecules that assemble into microfibrils, that in turn form fibrils (as in cartilage). Bone is formed of a heirarchy of microfibrils, fibrils and larger structures [Hartgerink et. al., 2001].

In current research, the lowest level in the heirarchical structure of bone has been simulated by synthesis of a peptide-apatite complex. Hartgerink and co-workers have synthesized an amphilic peptide where one end of the peptide is hydrophobic (composed of an alkyl chain) and the other end is hydrophilic (composed of the amino acid glycine). Functional groups for inter-peptide bonding and initiation of hydroxyapatite crystallization are also placed in the middle of the peptide molecular chain. The end of the chain also contains an amino acid sequence of Arginine, Glycine and Aspartine that are known to promote adhesion to cellular membranes. Strong adhesion between bone cells and their extracellular matrix is an important component in the strength and durability of the bone [Hargerink et. al., 2001].

To synthesize the peptide fibres, the peptide is dissolved in weakly alkaline water, which is then acidified to cause spontaneous assembly of peptide molecules into fibres of approximately 7 nm diameter and a length of the order of 5 micrometers. Crystallization of hydroxyapatite on the peptide fibers was achieved by irrigation with a mixture of aqueous calcium chloride and aqueous sodium hypophosphate. The small size of the fibres is believed to provide the optimum size of nucleation site to promote crystallization of the hydroxyapatite crystals (from reaction between calcium chloride and sodium hypophosphate).

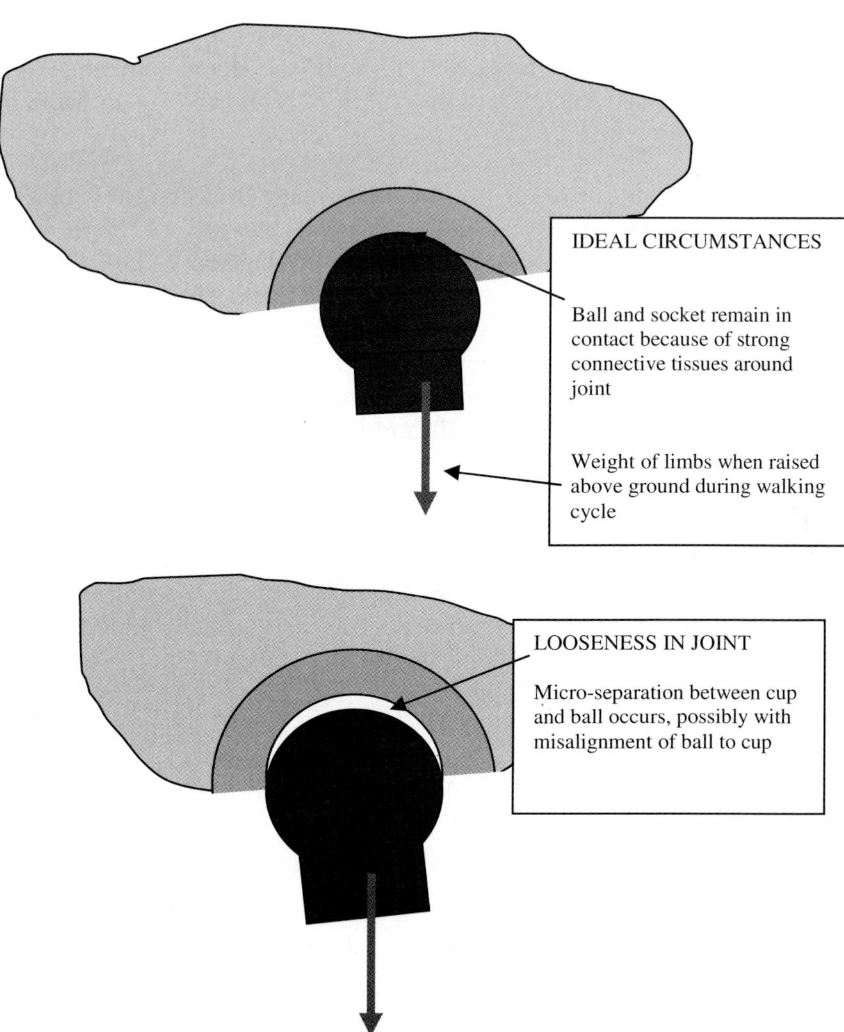

Fig 4.8. Micro-separation of implants and acceleration of wear.

While this research represents a very significant advance, only the smallest component of the bone structure has been simulated as noted by the researchers themselves. A complete bone has a complex heterogeneous structure, which is not static but grows and even atrophies in response to loading and patient health. There have also been some attempts to use biodegradable scaffolds such as poly-lactic acid in combination with reconstituted collagen, but these rely at least in part on natural materials (i.e. the collagen) whereas Hartgerink and co-workers have restricted themselves to synthetic materials.

4.7 Tissue inflammation and progressive bone resorption

4.7.1 *Tissue inflammations induced by wear particles of metals and polymers*

In machinery, wear not only consumes materials but also leads to the formation of wear debris, which may cause secondary problems. A similar yet more acute situation exists within human tissues surrounding the orthopaedic prosthesis. Of particular concern are metal particles and particles of UHMWPE because of the severe pathological response generated. The size range of UHMWPE wear particles is found to strongly influence the intensity of inflammation, with a size range of 0.3 to 10 micrometres generating the strongest response [Green et al., 1998]. The average size of wear particles from hip prostheses is approximately 0.7 micrometres [Elfick et al., 2002], while the average size of wear particles from knee prostheses is about 2 micrometres [Shanbhag et al. 2000]. The larger size of wear particles found in knee prostheses has been suggested as a reason for the lower incidence of inflammation in the knee prostheses as compared to the hip prosthesis [Shanbhag et al., 2000]. Reasons for the difference in average debris size are not fully understood. Metal wear particles, typically a few micrometres in size, may also generate a strong inflammation response from the immune system [Charlebois et al., 2002]. Macrophages and lymphocytes try to ingest the wear particles and the metabolic activity leads to solvation of metal ions. Inflammation involves secretion of strong oxidants such as hydroperoxide and hypochlorite, these are capable of reacting with metal to form dissolved cations. Since orthopaedic prostheses are made of chromium, cobalt and molybdenum, problems of toxicity and allergy may arise. With UHMWPE and other polymers such as PTFE, a more prolonged and so more harmful inflammation response occurs than with wear particles of ceramics [Xing et al., 2002]. This is probably because the polymer particles are less toxic to the macrophages, thus allowing the macrophages to remain active for longer periods of time and in greater numbers. It is found that the macrophages can engulf several polymer wear particles and still remain viable [Xing et al., 2002]. Wherever macrophages congregate in a tissue they cause inflammation both directly and indirectly by attracting other inflammatory cells from the immune system. Severe inflammation leads to joint pain, stiffness and in some cases, irreversible tissue damage [Charnley, 1961 & 1963]. A common effect is osteolysis where the macrophages and other cells of the immune system attack the bone adjacent to the prosthesis. This weakening of the bone by abnormal immune activity is termed aseptic loosening. The interface between the PMMA cement and bone is a critical site for osteolysis [Amstutz et al., 1998]. The PMMA cement is rarely able to bond the prosthesis perfectly to the bone. Instead there is some fretting movement between the bone and the cement or within the fissured cement itself. This causes the release of PMMA wear particles, which cause inflammation just like the wear particles from the prosthesis. Damage to the bone (osteolysis) causes loosening of the stem and eventual failure of the prosthesis [Amstutz et al., 1998]. The process of aseptic loosening of prosthesis has been modeled as a cascade process involving motion, wear, debris release, tissue inflammation and destruction of bone [Clarke et al., 1992]. This process is illustrated schematically in Figure 4.9.

4.7.2 *Progressive bone resorption by load shielding*

A basic feature of bone is its dynamic response to loading, which renders bone fundamentally different from wood. Typically, the elastic modulus of bone is approximately 10 times less than most high strength metals. This means the contact stresses around the stem of an orthopaedic prosthesis are highly localised, instead of being distributed by a more flexible material. The bone sustaining high contact stresses becomes stronger while the bone that is unloaded becomes weaker by a phenomenon known as resorption. Bone resorption progresses slowly to cause prosthesis failure after a few years service. Current research [Seeram et al., 2003] is directed at producing a biocompatible composite that has an elastic modulus closer to bone, i.e. in the range of 10 to 20 GPa. A major difficulty is that bone has a higher modulus than all known polymers, this necessitates the development of composite materials suitable for service lifetimes of 20 years or more.

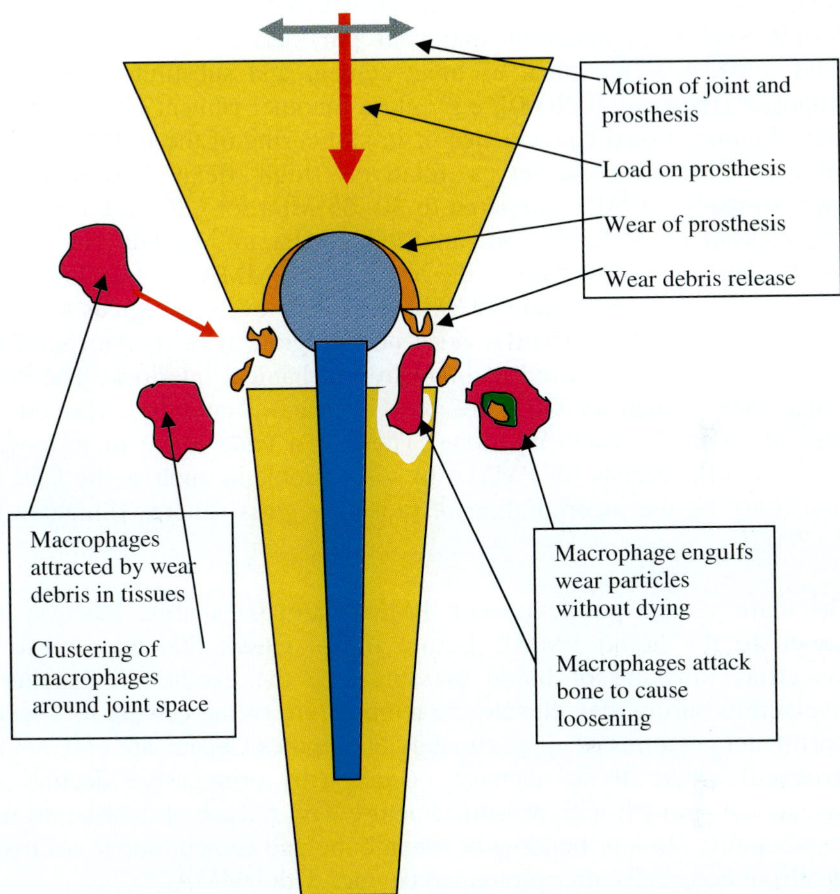

Fig 4.9. Mechanism of aseptic loosening of prosthesis when induced by large-scale release of wear debris.

4.7.3 *Cementation of orthopaedic prostheses to surrounding bone*

Bone cement is widely used to bond the stem of hip or knee prosthesis into the surrounding bone. The bone cement is typically made of Poly-Methyl-Meth-Acrylate Resin (PMMA), which is applied in liquid form during surgical implantation and later polymerizes to become a hard solid. PMMA is not ideal as bone cement and substitutes are being proposed [Higgs et al. 2000], e.g., glass ionomer cement [GIC]. Apart from the operational convenience of in-situ curing of the PMMA during surgery, PMMA possesses a relatively high flexural strength of approximately 70 MPa compared to 30- 35 MPa for GIC and a fracture toughness of 1.6 MPa.m$^{0.5}$ compared to 0.6 MPa. m$^{0.5}$ for GIC [Higges et al.]. Under suitable conditions, the bonding of PMMA to typical implant alloys such as TiAl6V4 and CoCrMo can reach levels as high as 40 MPa [Fischer et al., 2001]. PMMA does not integrate with the surrounding bone, instead it is believed to bond by mechanical interlock. The new replacements, such as GIC, are bioactive and would be expected to integrate with the enclosing bone. There is a wide range of proposed replacement materials for PMMA to solve problems such as the lack of bioactivity by the incorporation of bioactive glass spheres [Shinzato et al., 2002].

The main service problems with PMMA are; (i) allergic reaction by patient to the liquid PMMA before it has cured, this may cause a dangerous lowering of blood pressure, (ii) the exothermic reactions involved in curing may elevate the temperature of the cement to a level (curing temperatures of approximately 60 degrees Celsius are commonly observed) where tissue damage occurs, (iii) progressive decline in mechanical strength with possible fracture (iv) release of debris into the tissues and (v) loss of bonding between bone and cement due to necrosis (death) of bone cells after prolonged contact with PMMA.

If the initial problems of allergic response and excessive heat production are surpassed, then the loss of mechanical properties, debris release and loss of bonding become the life limiting factors.

4.7.3.1 <u>Loss of mechanical strength and resultant fracture</u>

The cement is subject to the same load oscillations as the implant itself and may fail by brittle fracture or by mechanical fatigue. Some authors [Murphy and Prendergast, 2001] consider that the mechanical fatigue resistance of the cement is the controlling factor on the life of the implant. The strength of the cement is strongly influenced by the level of porosity in the implant, since cracks are observed to be mainly initiated by pores and cavities [Murphy and Prendergast, 2001].

Acrylic bone cements are also prone to ageing, which would affect mechanical strength. Significant oxidative ageing of various commercial cements were found in hip implants but not knee implants. The main effect of ageing is to lower the molecular weight of the polymerized cement [Hughes et al., 2003].

4.7.3.2 <u>Debris release and inflammation of surrounding tissues</u>

In common with debris from the implant itself, debris from PMMA bone cement causes inflammation and a wider response from the immune system. It is found however that bone cement debris causes less stimulation of the immune system than do artificially generated PMMA particles [Miyaguchi et al., 2002]. PMMA particles are found to generate an immune response in mice but the nature of the response is not the same as other polymers [Tomazic-Jezic et al., 2001]. Wear debris from the used implant is found to generate a chronic immune response in patients [Farber et al. 2001] but it is not possible to distinguish the relative contributions of implant wear debris and cement debris. At any rate, the immune response to debris is closely associated with the phenomenon of aseptic loosening of the implant [Farber et al. 2001]. Aseptic loosening is a process where the implant and the surrounding bone become detached, without intervention by bacterial infection.

4.7.3.3 <u>Debonding of the cement to either the implant or the bone</u>

The bone cement has to bond both with the metal stem of the implant and with the surrounding bone. Both the metal-cement [Ohashi et al., 2001] and the bone-cement [Gough and Downes, 2001] interfaces are vulnerable to debonding. The physiological environment is found to be highly destructive to the metal-cement bond where destructive hydrolytic processes commonly occur [Ohashi et al., 2001]. An adhesion promoter can be added to the PMMA cement to try to prolong adhesion between metal and PMMA [Ohashi et al., 2001]. Another means of improving PMMA adhesion to the metal is to pretreat the metal surface of the implant with a silica/silane coating [Fischer et al, 2001].

Bonding of the PMMA cement to the bone is critically dependent on close contact between the adjacent bone cells and the solidified PMMA cement. The process of polymerization in PMMA is rarely complete and residual monomers remain, it is found that these monomers, e.g., tetrahydrofurfuryl methacrylate, is toxic to osteoblasts [bone cells] causing them to undergo apoptosis (cell death) [Gough and Downes, 2001].

A method of enhancing the bond between the PMMA cement and the surrounding bone is to produce a very rough surface on the bone in the implant socket. The PMMA then forms projections into the recesses on the bone surface (interdigitation), which then enhances the degree of mechanical interlock. The strengthening effect from this greatly extended mechanical interlock has been compared to the strengthening effect in a composite material [Lucksanasombool et al., 2003].

4.8 Bone fixation plates and spinal implants

4.8.1 *Fracture plates*

Complex or severe bone fractures, which are unlikely to heal by themselves, are often repaired with surgically fitted plates of stainless steel. The plates are held together by screws in an assembly that clamps the fractured bone. In most cases, these plates give reliable structural support with few instances of fracture. A major service problem is fretting corrosion between the screw-heads and the plate. Fretting is the microscopic reciprocating motion that occurs between clamped surfaces that sustain variable loads. The amplitude of the motion is exceedingly small, typically about 1 micrometre, but this is sufficient to cause what is termed fretting wear [Stachowiak and Batchelor, 2000]. As the user subjects the plates and screws to variable loads during normal limb motion, fretting wear occurs and metallic wear debris is released into the surrounding tissue. As discussed above, this metallic debris is inimical to human tissue, causing problems of inflammation and toxicity from dissolved metal ions such as chromium. Fretting although mechanical in origin is significantly accelerated by corrosion where the fretting movement efficiently fractures and expels brittle corrosion products from the wear scar. The saline environment around an implant is found to cause a significant acceleration of fretting wear in standard implant metal alloys such as 316L stainless steel, Co-Cr-Mo alloy and Ti-6Al-4V alloy [He et al., 2001]. Protein adsorption on the fretting surfaces (and all the other metal surfaces) modifies the fretting process and may accelerate fretting wear for some metals [Barril et al., 2002, Fu et al., 1999]. Earlier work by Merritt and Brown showed that common proteins such as albumen are found to increase the wear of iron but not of other metals such as copper.

Most structural metals, with the exception of magnesium discussed below, have an elastic modulus, which is significantly greater than bone. Cortical bone has an elastic modulus in the range of 7 to 25 GPa, with variation between different skeletal members and orientation within the bone. Most hard metals such as stainless and cobalt alloys have an elastic modulus of approximately 200 GPa, which is more than 10 times higher than that of bone. The high stiffness of structural metals causes parts of the bone around a plate clamp to become unloaded or 'shielded' from the load. The bone cells will atrophy unless subjected to mechanical stress and as a result of the load shielding; the bone around the clamp is often resorbed. A compromise is necessary between adequate clamp stiffness for short-term fracture healing and adequate load transfer to ensure maintenance of bone cell function [Seeram et al., 2003]. Polymer composites are being developed with high strength but a lower elastic modulus that is similar to bone. It is necessary to use a polymer composite rather than pure polymer because polymers have elastic moduli in the range of 1 to 10 GPa, which is too flexible for bone fixation [Seeram et al., 2003].

4.8.2 *Spinal implants*

Failure of intervertebral discs is a common cause of severe back pain, it is often ameliorated by the removal of the disc and fusion of adjacent vertebra by Discectomy (disc removal) and bone grafts. This is not an ideal solution because it compromises the flexiblity of the spine and causes a health problem known as Post Discectomy Syndrome [Zollner

2000]. A spinal implant, which satisfactorily serves as an inter-vertebral disc remains a subject of research, despite its practical importance. An initially offered solution involved metal balls, which were inserted in the space vacated by the disc. Metal balls provide a limited amount of elastic movement but will indent the contacting bone. Most work is now directed towards the use of compliant polymers and hydrogels, e.g. silicone elastomers and hydrogels [Bao et al., 2000 Ambrosio et al. 2000]. A recent development is the in-situ casting of poly-methyl-siloxane polymer (PMSO) in the space vacated by the disc [Zollner, 2000]. Mechanical testing of cadaver spines fitted with PMSO artificial discs reveals that the flexibility of an implanted spine is comparable to a healthy normal spine [Zollner, 2000]. The PMSO prosthesis does not appear to have yet been tested *in vivo* (in a living animal or human). The long-term service characteristics of this spinal implant remain unknown. A more recent development on the spinal implants include UHMWPE cylinders sandwiched between Ti discs to provide cushioning effect during compression due to flexion of spine.

Another form of prosthesis for the intervertebral disc is called the 'Rotocage', which is illustrated schematically in Figure 4.10.

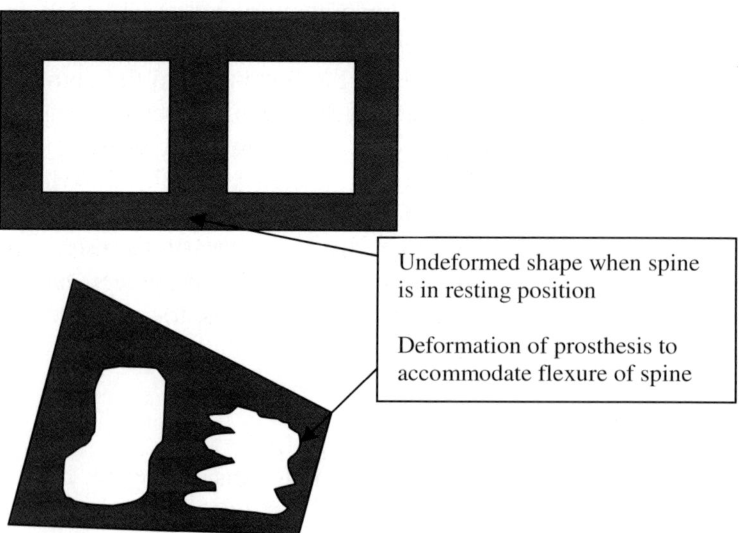

Fig 4.10. The Rotocage design of prosthesis for intervertebral disc, adapated from Toh et al. 2000.[Toh et al. 2000].

It is found that the Rotocage also offers a comparable flexibility to natural discs when fitted into a cadaver spine, but like the PMSO moulding, its long-term biocompatiblity remains unexplored [Toh et al. 2000].

4.9 Summary

There is a wide variety of orthopaedic implants in current use with two basic types of implant; plates and elastic supports to offer bone fixture, articulating implants to restore function of synovial joints. The articulating implants may be expected to suffer more from problems of wear than the fixture implants, but these also suffer from wear due to unintended microscopic movements within the implant and the adjacent bone. All orthopaedic implants have to be resistant to corrosion from bodily fluids. Bones and joints are sensitive to the leaching of toxins and irritants from implants, so the implant material must not only be robust but also be strictly biocompatible. Conversion of implant material to wear debris greatly increases its chance of causing harm to the body. In most cases, the sensitivity of the body to wear debris is more likely to cause failure of the implant rather than structural damage to the implant by wear.

References

L. Ambrosio, P.A. Netti, S. Iannace, S.J. Huang and L. Nicolais, Composite hydrogels for intervertebral disc prostheses, *Journal of Materials Science, Materials in Medicine*, 1996, Vol. 7, pp. 251-254.

H.C. Amstutz, P. Campbell, H. McKellop, T. P. Schmalzried, W.J. Gillespie, D. Howie, J. Jacbos, J. Medley and K. Merritt, Metal on Metal Total Hip Replacement Workshop Consensus Document, Clinical Orthopaedics and Related Research, 1996, Vol 329S (Supplement), pp. S297-S303.

H.C. Amstutz, P. Grigoris and F.J. Dorey, Evolution and future of surface replacement of the hip, Journal of Orthopaedic Science, 1998, Vol. 3, pp. 169-186.

Q.B. Bao, G.M. McCullen, P.A. Higham, J.H. Dumbleton and H.A. Yuan, The artificial disc: theory, design and materials, *Biomaterials*, 1996, Vol. 17, pp. 1157-1167.

G.C. Ballantine and G.W. Stachowiak, The effects of lipid depletion on osteoarthritic wear, Wear, 2002, Vol. 253, pp. 385-393.

S. Barril, N. Debaud, S. Mischler and D. Landolt, A tribo-chemical apparatus for in-vitro investigation of fretting-corrosion of metallic implant materials, Wear, 2002, Vol. 252, pp. 744-754.

A.W. Batchelor and G.W. Stachowiak, Arthritis and the interacting mechanisms of synovial joint lubrication. Part 1: Operating conditions and the environment, Journal of Orthopaedic Rheumatology, 1996, Vol. 9, pp. 3-10.

A.W. Batchelor and G.W. Stachowiak, Arthritis and the interacting mechanisms of synovial joint lubrication. Part 2: Joint lubrication and its relation to arthritis, Journal of Orthopaedic Rheumatology, 1996, Vol. 9, pp. 11-21.

A.W. Batchelor and M. Chandrasekaran, The role of proteins in synovial lubrication, Proc. 6th Int. Tribology Conf., AUSTRIB 2002, Perth, Western Australia, 2-5 Dec. 2002, publ. University of Western Australia, edit. G.W. Stachowiak, pp. 289-292.

A.A. Besong, J.L. Tipper, E. Ingham, M.H. Stone, B.M. Wroblewski and J. Fisher, Quantitative comparison of wear debris from UHMWPE that has and has not been sterilized by gamma radiation, Journal of Bone and Joint Surgery, 1998, Vol. 80B, pp. 340-344.

Jonathan Black, Metal on Metal Bearings: A practical alternative on polyethylene total joints?, Clinical Orthopaedics and Related Research, 1996, Vol. 329S (Supplement), pp. S244-255.

J. Blamey, S. Rajan, R. Dawber, A. Unsworth (1991). Compliant prosthesis for hip joints. J. Bone Joint Surg. **73-B**: Supp 1.

M. Bohler, Y. Mochida, Th. W. Bauer, H. Plenk and M. Salzer, Wear debris from two different alumina-on-alumina total hip arthroplasties, Journal of Bone and Joint Surgery, 2000, Vol. 82B, No. 6, pp. 901-909.

W.G. Brodbeck, J. Patel, G. Voskerician, E. Christenson, M.S. Shive, Y. Nakayama, T. Matsuda, N.P. Ziats and J.M. Anderson, Biomaterial adherent macrophage apoptosis is increased by hydrophilic and anionic substrates in vivo, Proceedings of the National Academy of Sciences, USA, published on line, doi: 10.1073/pnas162124199.

R.A. Buchanan, E.D. Rigney, J.M. Williams, Ion implantation of surgical Ti6Al4V for improved resistance to wear-accelerated corrosion, Journal of Biomedical Materials research, 1987, Vol. 21, 355-366.

Patrick A. Campbell, Mark Wang, Harlan C. Amstutz and Stuart B. Goodman, Positive cytokine production in failed metal-on-metal total hip replacements, Acta Orthopaedica Scandinavica, 2002, Vol. 73, No. 5, pp. 506-512.

S.J. Charlebois, A.U. Daniels and R.A. Smith, Metabolic heat production as a measure of macrophage response to particles from orthopaedic implant materials, Journal of Biomedical Materials Research, 2002, Vol. 59, No. 1, pp. 166-175.

J.C. Charnley, Arthroplasty of the hip: A new operation, The Lancet, 1961, I, pp. 1129-32.

J.C. Charnley, Tissue reactions to polytetrafluoroethylene, The Lancet, 1963, II, p.1379.

I.C. Clarke, P. Campbell and N. Kossovsky, Debris-mediated osteolysis – A cascade phenomenon involving motion, wear, particulates, macrophage induction and bone lysis. In: K.R.S. John (editor), Particulate debris from medical implants: Mechanisms of formation and biological consequences, Philadelphia: American Society for Testing and Materials, 1992, pp. 7-26.

C. Cooper, Occupational activity and the risk of osteoarthritis, Journal of Rheumatology, 1995, Vol. 22, No. 43, pp. 10-12.

O.H. Craciunescu, L.E. Howle and S.T. Clegg, Experimental evaluation of the thermal properties of two tissue equivalent phantom materials, International Journal of Hyperthermia, 1999, Vol. 15, pp. 509-518

W.G. Di Maio, W.B. Lilly, W.C. Moore and K.A. Saum, Low wear, low oxidation radiation crosslinked UHMWPE, 1998, Transactions of the 44th Orthopedic Research Society, 23:328.

P.F. Doorn, P.A. Campbell, J. Worrall, P.D. Benya, H.A. McKellop and H.C. Amstutz, Metal wear particle characterization from metal on metal total hip replacements: Transmission electron microscopy study of periprosthetic tissues and isolated particles, Journal of Biomedical Materials Research, 1998, Vol. 42, No. 1, pp. 103-111.

J.H. Dumbleton, Tribology of natural and artificial joints, Elsevier, 1981, Amsterdam.

C.H. Evans, The role of proteinases in cartilage destruction, Agents and Actions, Supplements, 1991, Vol. 32, pp. 135-152.

A.P.D. Elfick, S.M. Green, S. Krikler and A. Unsworth, The nature and dissemination of UHMWPE wear debris retrieved from periprosthetic tissue of THR, Journal of Biomedical Materials Research, Part A, 2003, No. 1, pp. 95-108.

A. Farber, R. Chin, Y. Song, P. Huie, S. Goodman, Chronic antigen-specific immune system activation may potentially be involved in the loosening of cemented acetabular components, Journal of Biomedical Materials Research, 2001, Vol. 55, No. 3, pp. 433-441.

H. Fischer, D.C. Wirtz, M. Weber, M. Neuss, F.U. Niethard and R. Marx, Improvement of the long-term adhesive strength between metal stem and polymethylmethacrylate bone cement by a silica/silane interlayer system, Journal of Biomedical Materials Research, 2001, Vol. 57, No. 3, pp. 413-418.

Y. Fu, A.W. Batchelor and K.A. Khor, Fretting wear behavior of thermal sprayed hydroxyapatite coating lubricated with bovine albumin, Wear, 1999, Vol. 230, pp. 98-102.

R.S. Gates, S.M. Hsu, E.E. Klaus, Tribochemical mechanism of alumina with water, Tribology Transactions, 1989, Vol. 32, pp. 357-363.

J.E. Gough and S. Downes, Osteoblast cell death and methacrylate polymers involves apoptosis, Journal of Biomedical Materials Research, 2001, Vol. 57, No. 4, pp. 497-505.

T.R. Green, J. Fisher, M. Stone, B.M. Wroblewski and E. Ingham, Polyethylene particles of a 'critical size' are necessary for the induction of cytokines by macrophages in vitro', Biomaterials, 1998, 19(24), pp. 2297-22302.

Jeffrey.D. Hartgerink, Elia. Beniash and Samuel.I. Stupp, Self-assembly and mineralization of peptide-amphiphile nanofibers, Science, 2001(Nov. 23rd), Vol. 294, pp. 1684-1693.

B. Hastings, D. Huston, E. Reber and W. Di Maio, Knee wear testing of a radiation cross-linked and remelted UHMWPE, Transactions of the 25th Society for Biomaterials, 1999, 22:328.

D. He, T. Zhang and Y. Wu, Mechanisms responsible for synergy between fretting and corrosion for three biomaterialsin saline solution, Wear, 2001, Vol. 250, pp. 180-187.

Larry L. Hench, The story of bioglass (trademark): from concept to clinic, in Imperial College Inaugural Lectures in Materials Science and Engineering, edit. Don W. Pashley, Imperial College Press, 2001, London, United Kingdom, pp. 203-229.

W.A.J. Higgs, P.Lucksanasombool, R.J.E.D. Higgs and M.V. Swain, Characterization of a new bioactive bone cement, a comparison with PMMA, Poster Session –Biomaterials – Valencia D, 46th Annual Meeting, Orthopaedic Research Society, 12-15 March, 2000, Orlando, Florida, USA.

B.A. Hills and B.D. Butler, Identification of surfactants in synovial fluid and their ability to act as boundary lubricants, Annals of the Rheumatic Diseases, 1984, Vol. 48, pp. 51-57.

K.F. Hughes, M.D. Ries, L.A. Pruitt, Structural degradationof acrylic bone cements due to in vivo and simulated aging, Journal of Biomedical Materials Research, Part A, 2003, Vol. 65A, No. 2, pp. 126-135.

K. Imado, A. Miura, H. Miyagawa, T. Harran and H. Higaki, The effects of frictional heat on mechanical property and wear rate of UHMWPE for use in artificial joints, Proc. 10th International Conference on Biomedical Engineering, 6-9 Dec. 2000, Singapore, edit. JCH Goh, publ. National University of Singapore, pp. 215-216.

E.W. Lee and H.T. Kim, Early fatigue failures of cemented, forged, cobalt-chromium femoral stems at the neck-shoulder junction, The Journal of Arthroplasty, 2001, Vol. 16, No. 2, pp. 236-238.

T.J. Joyce, C. Rieker and A. Unsworth, In Vitro wear testing of metal-on-polymer metacarpophalangeal prostheses, Proc. Int. Tribology Conf., AUSTRIB '02, Perth, Australia, 2-5 December 2002, editor G.W. Stachowiak, publ. University of Western Australia, Vol. 1, pp. 323-329.

A.G. Kay, J.V. Lieffs and J.T. Scott, Experience with silastic prostheses in the rheumatoid hand: a 5 year follow up, Annals of the Rheumatic Diseases, 1978, Vol. 37, pp. 255-258.

T. B. Kirk, A.S. Wilson and G.W. Stachowiak, The morphology and composition of the superficial zone of mammalian articular cartilage, Journal of Orthopaedic Rheumatology, 1993, Vol. 6, pp. 21-28.

H.K. Koerten, J.J.M. Onderwater, E.W.A. Koerten, F.P. Bernoski, and R.G.H.H. Nelissen, Observations at the articular surface of hip prostheses: An analytical electron microscopy study on wear and corrosion, Journal of Biomedical Materials Research, 2001, Vol. 54, No. 4, pp. 591-596.

S.M.Kurtz, O.K. Muratoglu, M. Evans and A.A. Edidin, Advances in the processing, sterilization and cross-linking of ultra-high molecular weight polyethylene for total joint arthroplasty, Biomaterials, 1999, Vol. 20, pp. 1659-1688.

S.W.K. Kweh, K.A. Khor and P. Cheang, Plasma-sprayed hydroxyapatite (HA) coatings with flame-spheroidized feed stock: Microstructure and mechanical properties, Biomaterials, 2000, Vol. 21, pp. 1223-1234

S. Leeuwenburgh, J. Wolke, J. Schoonman and J. Jansen, Electrostatic spray deposition (ESD) of calcium phosphate coatings, Journal of Biomedical Materials Research Part A, 2003, Vol. 66A, No. 2, pp. 330-334.

T. Little, M.A.R. Freeman and S.A.R. Swanson, Experiments on friction in the human hip joint, Lubrication and Wear in Joints, Proc. Symposium organized by the Biological Engineering Society, editor, Vernon Wright, Leeds, London, Sector, Lippincott Publisher, Philadelphia, USA, 17th April 1969, pp. 110-114.

P.Lucksanasombool, W.A.J. Higs, M. Ignat, R.J.E.D. Higgs and M.V. Swain, Comparison of failure characteristics of a range of cancellous bone-bone cement composites, Journal of Biomedical Materials Research, Part A, 2003, Vol. 64A, pp. 93-104.

J.D. Mabrey, A. Afsar-Keshmiri, G.A. McGlung II, M.A. Pember, T.M. Wooldridge and C.M. Agrawal, Comparison of UHMWPE particles in synovial fluid and tissues from failed THA, Journal of Biomedical Materials, 2001, Vol. 58, No. 2, pp. 196-202.

M. Maiotti, G. Monteleone, U. Tarantino, G.F. Fasciglione, S. Marini and M. Coletta, Correlation between osteoarthritic cartilage damage and levels of proteinases and proteinase inhibitors in synovial fluid for the knee joint, Arthroscopy, 2000, Vol. 16, No. 5, pp. 522-526.

H. Malchau and P. Herberts, Prognosis of total hip replacement, Revision and re-revision rate in THR: a revision risk study of 148,359 primary operations, 65th Annual Meeting of the American Academy of Orthopaedic Surgeons (Scientific Exhibition), 19-23 February, 1998, New Orleans, USA.

V. Maquet, A.R. Boccaccini, L. Pravata, I. Notinger and R. Jerome, Preparation, characterization and in vitro degradation of bioresorbable and bioactive composites based on Bioglass (Trademark) filled polylactide foams, Journal of Biomedical Materials Research, Part A, 2003, Vol. 66A, No. 2, pp. 35-346.

A. Maroudas, Balance between swelling pressure and collagen tension in normal and degenerate cartilage, Nature, 1976, Vol. 260, pp. 808-809.

D. Mazzucco and M. Spector, Effects of contact area and stress on the volumetric wear of ultrahigh molecular weight polyethylene, Wear, 2003, Vol. 254, pp. 514-522.

C.W. McCutchen, Sponge-hydrostatic and weeping bearings, Nature, 1959, Vol. 184, page 1284.

B.K. Milthorpe, Hydroxyapatite based materials for replacement of bone in load bearing situations, Proc. 10th International Conference on Biomedical Engineering, Singapore, edit. JCH Goh, publ. National University of Singapore, 6-9 Dec. 2000, Singapore, pp. 38-39.

M. Miyaguchi, A. Kobayashi, H. Iwaki, H. Ohashi, Y. Kadoya and Y. Yamano, Human monocyte response to retrieved polymethylmethacrylate particles, Journal of Biomedical Materials Research, 2002, Vol. 62, No. 3, pp. 331-337.

Y. Morita, K. Nakata and K. Ikeuchi, Wear properties of zirconia/alumina combination for joint prostheses, Wear, 2003, Vol. 254, pp. 147-153.

V.C. Mow, The role of lubrication in biomechanical joints, Transactions of the ASME, Journal of Lubrication Technology, 1969, Vol. 91, pp.320-329.

O.K. Muratoglu, C.R. Bragdon, D.O. O'Connor, M. Jasty and W.H. Harris, A novel method of cross-linking ultra-high-molecular weight polyethylene to improve wear, reduce oxidation and retain mechanical properties, Recipient of the 1999 HAP Paul Award, Journal of Arthroplasty, 2001, Vol. 16, pp. 149-160.

O.K. Muratoglu, C.R. Bragdon, D.O. O'Connor, R.S. Perinchief, J.T. Travers, M. Jasty, H.E. Rubash and W.H. Harris, Markedly improved adhesive wear and delamination resistance with a highly crosslinked UHMWPE for use in total knee arthroplasty, Transactions of the 27th Annual Meeting of the Society for Biomaterials, 2001, 24:29.

B.P. Murphy and P.J. Prendergast, The relationship between stress, porosity, and non-linear damage accumulation in acrylic bone cement, Journal of Biomedical Materials Research, 2002, Vol. 59, No. 4, pp. 646-654.

P.L. O'Neill and G.W. Stachowiak, The inverse thixotropic behaviour of synovial fluid and its relation to the lubrication of synovial joints, Journal of Orthopaedic Rheumatology, 1996, Vol. 9, pp. 222-228.

P.L. O'Neill, G.W. Stachowiak and G.J. Carroll, The elastohydrodynamic properties of arthritic synovial fluid, Journal of Orthopaedic Rheumatology, 1989, Vol. 2, pp. 219-230.

K.L. Ohashi, S.A. Yerby and R.H. Dauskardt, Effects of an adhesion promoter on the debond resistance of a metal-polymethacrylate interface, Journal of Biomedical Materials Research, 2001, Vol. 54, No. 3, pp. 419-427.

H. Oonishi, Y. Kadoya and S. Masuda, Gamma-irradiated cross-linked polyethylene in total hip replacements - analysis of retrieved sockets after long-term implantation, Journal of Biomedical Materials Research, 2001, Vol. 58, No. 2, pp. 167-171.

I.G. Otterness, M.L. Bliven, J.D. Eskra, J.M. te Koppele, H.A. Stukenbrok and A.-J. Milici, Cartilage damage after intraarticular exposure to collagenase 3, Osteoarthritis and Cartilage, 2000, Vol. 8, pp. 366-373.

R.S. Pascaud, W.T. Evans, P.J.J. McCullagh and D.P. Fitzpatrick, Influence of gamma- irradiation sterilization and temperature on the fracture toughness of Ultra-High-Molecular-Weight Polyethylene, Biomaterials, 1997, Vol. 18, pp. 727-735.

Jody Redepenning, Guhanand Venkataram, Jun Chen and Nathan Stafford, Electrochemical preparation of chitosan/hydroxyapatite composite coatings on titanium surfaces, Journal of Biomedical Materials Research Part A, 2003, Vol. 66A, No.2, pp. 411-416.

L. Savarino, D. Granchi, G. Ciapetti, E. Cenni, M. Greco, R. Rotini, C.A.Vernosesi, N. Baldini and A. Giunti, Ion release in stable hip arthroplasties using metal-on-metal articulating surfaces: A comparison between short-term and long-term results, Journal of Biomedical Materials Research, Part A, 2003, Vol. 66A, No. 3, pp. 450-456.

L. Savarino, M. Fini, G. Ciapetti, E. Cenni, D. Granchi, N. Baldini, M. Greco, G. Rizzi, R. Giardino and A. Giunti, Biologic effects of surface roughness and fluorhydroxyapatite coating on osteointegration in external fixation systems: An *in vivo* experimental study, Journal of Biomedical Materials Research, Part A, 2003, Vol. 66A, No. 3, pp. 652-661.

Seeram Ramakrishna, Z-M. Huang and G.V. Kumar, J. Meyer and A.W. Batchelor, Introduction to Biocomposites, Imperial College Press, 2004 (in preparation).

T.P. Schmalzfried and J.J. Callaghan, Wear in total hip and knee replacements, Journal of Bone and Joint Surgery, 1999, Vol. 81A, No. 1, pp. 115-136.

I.M. Schwarz and B.A. Hills, Surface-active phospholipid as the lubricating component of lubricin, British Journal of Rheumatology, 1998, Vol. 37, pp. 21-26.

Richard Shalak and Shu Chien (editors), Handbook of bioengineering, Publ.. McGraw Hill, New York, 1987.

A.S. Shanbhag, H.O. Bailey, D.-S. Hawng, C.W. Cha, N.G. Eror and H.E. Rubash, Quantitative analysis of ultrahigh molecular weight polyethylene (UHMWPE) wear debris associated with total knee replacements, Journal of Biomedical Materials Research, 2000, Vol. 53, No. 1, pp. 100-110.

S. Shinzato, T. Nakamura, T. Kokubo and Y. Kitamura, PMMA-based bioactive cement: Effect of glass bead filler content and histological change with time, Journal of Biomedical Materials Research, 2002, Vol. 59, No. 2, pp. 225-232.

H.-P.Sieber, C.B. Rieker and P. Kottig, Analysis of 118 second-generation metal-on-metal retrieved hip implants, The Journal of Bone and Joint Surgery (British), 1999, Vol. 81, No. B1, pp. 46-50.

G.W. Stachowiak, A.W. Batchelor, and L.J. Griffiths, Friction and wear changes in synovial joints, Wear, 1994, Vol. 171, pp. 135-142.

G.W. Stachowiak and A.W. Batchelor, Engineering Tribology, 2nd edition, Butterworth-Heinemann, 2000, Woburn, MA, USA.

G.W. Stachowiak, Private communication, Nov. 1995.

T.D. Stewart, J.L. Tipper, G. Insley, R.M. Streicher, E. Ingham and J. Fisher, Long-term wear of ceramic matrix composite materials for hip prostheses under severe swing phase microseparation, Journal of Biomedical Materials Research, Part B: Applied Biomaterials, 2003, Vol. 66B, pp. 567-573.

D.A. Swann, E.L. Radin, M. Nazimiec, P.A. Weisser, N. Curran and G. Lewinnek, Role of hyaluronic acid in joint lubrication, Annals of the Rheumatic Diseases, 1974, Vol. 33, pp. 318-326.

D.A. Swann, R.B. Hendren, E.L. Radin, S.L. Sotman and E.A. Duda, The lubricating activity of synovial fluid glycoproteins, Arthritis and Rheumatism, 1981, Vol. 24, No. 1, pp. 22-30.

A.B. Swanson, Flexible implant arthroplasty for arthritic finger joints, Journal of Bone and Joint Surgery, 1972, Vol. 54A, pp. 435-455.

Eric Swarts, Susan J. Miller, Cathie V. Keogh, Gerald Lim and Richard J. Beaver Fractured Whiteside Ortholoc II knee components, The Journal of Arthoplasty, Fractured Whiteside Ortholoc knee components. The Journal of Arthroplasty, 2001, Vol. 16, No. 7, pp. 927-934.

S. Tanaka, C. Hamanishi, H. Kikuchi and K. Fukuda, factors related to degradation of articular cartilage in osteoarthritis: a review, Seminars in Arthritis and Rheumatism, 1998, Vol. 27, No. 6, pp. 392-399.

S.L. Toh, J.C.H. Goh, H.K. Wong and W.J. Koh, Biomechanical evalution of the rotocage PLIF device, Proc. 10th International Conference on Biomechanical Engineering, 6-9 Dec. 2000, Singapore, edit. JCH Goh, publ. National University of Singapore, pp. 360-361.

J.L. Tipper, E. Ingham, J.L. Hailey, A.A. Besong, J. Fisher, B.M. Wroblewski and M. Stone, Quantitative analysis of polyethylene wear debris, wear rate and head damage in retrieved Charnley hip prostheses, Journal of Materials Science: Materials in Medicine, 2000, Vol. 11, No. 2, pp. 117-124.

V.J. Tomazic-Jezic, Katharine Merritt and T.H. Umbriet, Significance of the type and the size of biomaterial particles on phagocytosis and tissue distribution, Journal of Biomedical Materials Research, 2001, Vol. 55, No. 4, pp. 523-529.

A. Unsworth, D. Dowson and V. Wright, Frictonal behaviour of human synovial joints – 1., Natural joints, Transactions of the ASME, Journal of Lubrication technology, 1975, Vol. 97, No. 3, pp. 377-382.

A. Unsworth, M.J. Pearcy, E.F.T. White and G. White (1987). "Soft layer lubrication of artificial hip joints". Proceedings of the Institution of Mechanical Engineers International Conference Volume on Tribology. London, June 1987, pp 715-724

A Unsworth. Compliant layer lubrication. Keynote Address. Proceedings of the 5th Australian International Tribology Conference, Brisbane, Australia, (AUSTRIB), December 1998.248-255, edit. D. Hargreaves.

C.J.M. Van Loon, M.A. Wisse, M.C. de Waal Malefijt, R.H. Jansen and R.P.H. Veth, The kinematic total knee arthroplasty, a 10 to 15 year follow-up and survival analysis, Arch. Orthop Trauma Surg, 2000, Vol. 120, pp. 48-52.

M.L. Villarraga, S.M. Kurtz, M.P. Herr and A.A. Edidin, Multi-axial fatigue behavior of conventional and highly crosslinked UHMWPE during cyclic small punch testing, Journal of Biomedical Materials Research Part A, 2003, Vol. 66A, No. 2, pp. 298-309.

A.Webb, G.W. Stachowiak, P.L. O'Neill and A.W. Batchelor, The effects of temperature changes and arthritis on the lubricating properties of synovial fluid, Journal of Orthopaedic Rheumatology, 1993, Vol. 6, pp. 81-86.

D.F. Williams, Review-Tissue biomaterial interactions, Journal of Materials Science, 1987, Vol. 22, pp. 3421-3445.

P.F. Williams III, G.L. Powell and M. LaBerge, Sliding friction analysis of phosphatidylcholine as a boundary lubricant for articular cartilage, Proceedings of the Institute of Mechanical Engineers, Part H: Journal of Engineering in Medicine, 1993, Vol. 207, pp. 59-66.

S. Xing, J.P. Santerre, R.S. Labow and E.L. Boynton, The effect of polyethylene particle phagocytosis on the viability of mature human macrophages, Journal of Biomedical Materials Research Part A, Vol. 61, No. 4, 2002, pages 619-627.

Jan Zollner, A 3-Dimensional Biomechanical investigation of a new type of artificial lumbar disc, Proc. 10th International Conference on Biomechanical Engineering, 6-9 Dec. 2000, Singapore, edit. JCH Goh, publ. National University of Singapore, pp. 73-74.

Chapter 5

Cardiac, Vascular and Neural Implants

5.1 Introduction

Numerous articles have been devoted to describing either the high prevalence of heart disease around the world or else possible strategies to reduce heart disease. Much research is devoted to the development of new treatment methods for patients with heart disease. A recent example is the announcement of a technique to grow human arteries in vitro from cells collected either from the patient or from a suitable donor [Pilcher, 2003]. While externally grown segments of arteries may become an invaluable material for the repair of ischaemic heart disease and thrombosis else in the human body, implants of non-living material such as artificial heart valves still have a vital role in medical treatment. The durability of the implant and the minimum of undesirable side effects, such as e.g., damage to red blood cells remains the subject of much research.

Cardiac implants are a rapidly developing area of surgery with new forms of implants continuously being developed. These implants are expected to survive and provide a longer and better quality of life than conventional treatments, which include pharmacologic or transplants. In most cases the cardiac implants are semi-permanent or permanent. The most important prerequisite of such implant is its ability to fit into the system for which it has been designed in terms of volume, mass, gender and age etc., with minimal or no adverse impact on the pathology.

107

Adverse impact generated may vary from patient to patient depending on the gender, pathologic conditions and the age.   In addition to these requirements the heat transfer requirements are to be met by the designed implant [Rosenverg]. Currently a new type of degradable cardiac implant based on magnesium alloys is being developed [Haferkampf et al., 2000]. Magnesium displays low toxicity to the human body and is rapidly corroded by saline solutions. The density and elastic modulus of magnesium are closely comparable to bone.   The corrosion rate of magnesium can be controlled by alloying and by thermo-mechanical treatment. A significant problem with the use of magnesium that remains to be addressed is the replacement of aluminium as an alloying element since aluminium is very toxic. It is also necessary to achieve both sufficient ductility and corrosion resistance.

5.2   The origins and modes of heart disorder

Heart disease has become a very common health problem and is observed to associate with a diet high in animal fats and a lack of physical exercise. Genetic factors contribute greatly to the susceptibility of individuals to heart disease.   There are many modes of heart disorder, ranging from congenital defects and bacterial or viral infections to the widely discussed problems of ageing.

Cardiac health problems where implants may be used during medical treatment, mainly involve the heart valves and the heart muscle. Competent performance by the heart depends on precise control of blood flow by the heart valves. When a heart valve becomes leaky, reverse flow of blood will occur. This is known as regurgitation and is a form of heart disease. There are a variety of causes for heart valve leakage, many problems occur at the mitral valve where the blood flow is most intense. A common disorder of the mitral valve is stenosis, which is thickening of the valve flaps, typically after the deposition of scar tissue from an infection. Stenosis deprives the mitral valve flaps of the required flexibility to open and close at normal blood pressures. As a result, the blood pressure rises in order to ensure mitral valve opening. Another mitral valve disorder is prolapse where the valve flaps lose rigidity and are unable to close.

Heart muscle (myocardium) is very active and requires an adequate oxygen supply at all times. Blockage of the blood supply to the heart muscle, (myocardial ischaemia) causes pain and in severe cases, destruction of a portion of the heart muscle (myocardial infarction). Blockage of the cardiac blood vessels is often caused by arteriosclerosis, which is a gradual hardening and constriction of arterial walls. Arterial wall constriction is believed to be caused by deposits of cholesterol originating from the animal fat component of the human diet. Destruction of any part of the myocardium is permanent unless treated because of the inability of heart muscle cells to be replaced. A new development in biomaterials is the development of a patch of heart muscle based on a culture of heart muscle cells in a disposable scaffold. This type of cardiac prosthesis is discussed in later chapters.

5.3 Artificial heart valves

Artificial heart valves are either made out of entirely artificial materials such as pyrolytic carbon and titanium alloys, or are manufactured from denatured animal cardiac tissues. The various types of heart valve in current use are classified schematically in Figure 5.1

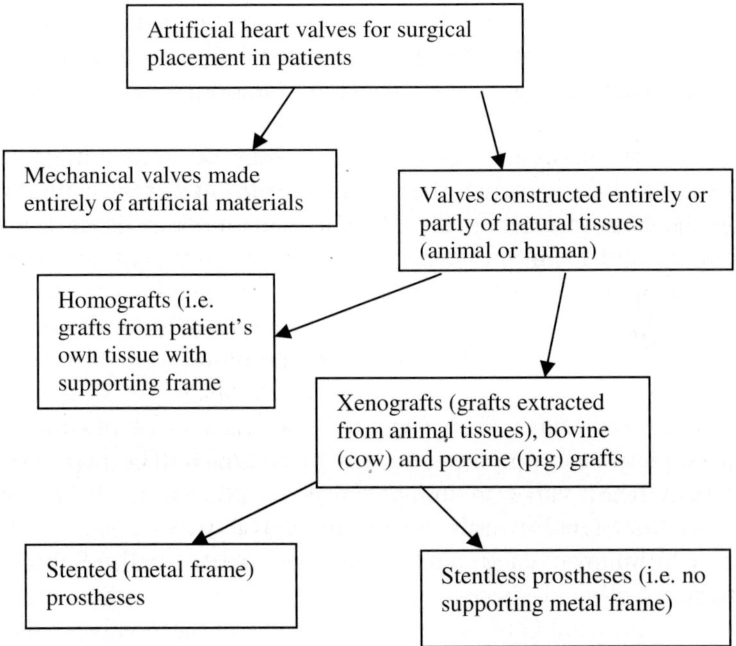

Fig 5.1. Classification of artificial heart valves according to origin.

5.3.1 *Valves made from artificial materials*

As highlighted in the introduction an artificial heart assist device would have certain requirements with respect to its biocompatibility, functionality and other standards such as electromagnetic interference and susceptibility. Biocompatibility described in the earlier sections of this book refers to minimal or no effects on the immune system of the body in addition to not promoting any infection, calcification or tissue necrosis. In terms of functionality a heart pump's performance is measured in terms of the cardiac output range. This varies from person to person who has been implanted with the heat assist device such as age, gender and other pathologic conditions. A typical example of such requirement for a 70 Kg person would be approximately 70 ml/min/Kg as resting cardiac output which totals to about 5 l/min and can go up to 8 l/min with light exercise. Maintenance of physiologic inlet and outlet pressures should be within the specified range, which depends on various factors relating to the patient. Besides this there should be a balance of pressure between the left and right pumps failing which it may result in pulmonary congestion (differential pressure shooting above 20 mm Hg). The device should also be able to adjust the cardiac output depending on the requirements of the patient. The nature of the tubes, conduits or connectors such as hard, soft, rough or smooth must be considered besides the volume and mass of such devices so as to not cause any damage to surrounding tissues or organs. Another requirement of such devices are to have matching heat transfer rates to that of natural organs so that the heat transfer to the blood or surrounding tissue are within basic limits under chronic basis. This latter requirement of comparable heat transfer applies more to cardiac assist devices ('pacemakers') than to the current design of heart valves. A possible future design of self-powered heart valve could involve heat release.

Various materials have been used for construction of prosthetic heart valves ranging from polymers, metals to ceramics. The first successful mechanical heart valve in humans was introduced in 1961 and was known as the Starr-Edwards caged half valve. It was made of Stellite (Cobalt-Chromium) cage with silicone rubber ball. Subsequently following its clinical success, other materials such as Titanium alloys, Pyrolytic carbon and hard ceramic were used. In these valves, the cages were mainly made of of Titanium alloys while the Pyrolytic carbon or hard ceramic were used as balls. A typical disadvantage of these valves included excessive noise and wearing of the struts by the ball and they were soon abandoned while the silicone ball is still in clinical use. An alternative to the caged design included the Wada-Cutter valve, which had a tilting design with a ring of Titanium and a disc of Polytetrafluoroethylene (PTFE). One of the problems with this type of valve was the excessive wear of the PTFE disc resulting in disc escape for a few patients. The PTFE was replaced in later designs with Pyrolytic carbon and the valve was further modified to overcome insufficient flushing leading to thrombosis. This valve known as the Medtronic-Hall valve has two projecting strut to retain the disc in place. A typical design of the valve is shown in Figure 5.2. The excellent biocompatibility of Pyrolytic carbon is the main reason for its wide use in the construction of heart valves. The most popular type of heart valve, the St Jude valve, contains two leaflets (similar to valve flaps) made of pyrolytic carbon. This material is comparatively weak, so it is often reinforced with metal frames made of titanium or cobalt alloys. Textiles made from artificial fibres such as polyester or PTFE, are used on the exterior of the valve where it contacts the heart tissue. The most common types of mechanical heart valve used today are made of pyrolytic carbon in titanium or carbon housings with a bi-leaflet configuration.

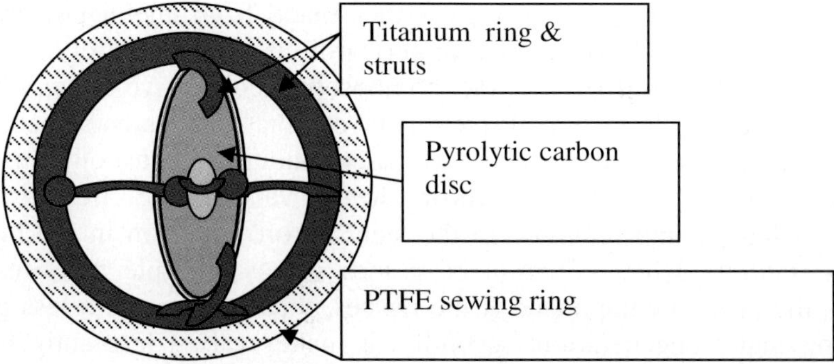

Fig 5.2.   A typical schematic model of Medtronic-Hall heart valve prosthesis (aortic version). *[adapted from C.Olin]*

5.3.1.1   Valves made from denatured animal tissues

An alternative to the mechanical heart valve is the use of naturally occurring valves. This is due to the problems associated with mechanical valves such as the need for life-long anticoagulation therapy and accompanying problems of bleeding. These can be classified into either homograft (from another member of the same species) or a xenograft, which is tissue taken from another species [Yoganathan; Cox-Gad; Schmidt and Baier]. Common sources of xenografts are the cow (bovine xenografts) and the pig (porcine xenografts). A typical problem associated with the use of cadaveric allografts is that they are no longer living tissue and lack the ability of cellular regeneration. This makes them vulnerable to degradation and calcification during long-term use. An alternative approach to overcome this lacuna was the placement of treated animal tissues on a rigid frame. These valves are termed as bioprosthetic heart valves and have been used successfully for about 45 years.   Bioprosthetic heart valves are available in a stented configuration whereas tissue valves are mounted on a rigid polymeric frame. Recently, there has been a great interest in the development of stentless heart valves, which include a large portion of aortic segment of xenograft in the design. Such stent-less valves have better haemodynamics (blood flow dynamics) and larger orifice area for a given size as compared to stented heart valves.

Aortic heart valve prostheses are either made from chemically treated porcine (pig) heart valve or bovine pericardium. The pericardium can be approximately described as a sac, composed of connective tissue with an inner lubricating layer of cells (serous layer), that surrounds the heart and allows it to pulsate without excessive frictional drag against other tissues. The tissue, e.g., porcine aortic heart valves, are treated with glutaraldehyde and mounted in the stent before insertion in the human body. Gluteraldehyde fixation of tissues serves multiple purposes. It fixes the protein component of the tissues, thus making them less prone to enzymatic degeneration; secondly, it makes valves less antigenic, it also sterilizes tissues. Tissue fixation is a form of cross-linking between protein molecules or other large molecules, especially in the extra-cellular matrix. Antigenic means to function as an antigen, which activates the immune system.

A major problem of porcine aortic bioprostheses (animal tissues adopted for use in humans) is calcification, which is the formation of hard calcium rich deposits on the valve surfaces. It is found that immersion of the porcine tissues in 80% ethanol suppresses calcification [Vyavahare et al., 1997; Lee et al., 1998]. Another method is to treat the porcine tissue with sulfonated PEO to reduce calcification or 2-amino oleic acid [Chen et al., 1994]. The ability of ethanol to dissolve and thereby remove lipids in the porcine tissue as well as cause changes in the collagen conformation is believed to be responsible for reduced calcification. The causes of pathological calcification of porcine heart valves are poorly understood. There are two possible mechanisms of calcification. The first one, widely cited, is hypothesized to result from glutaraldehyde-induced cellular "devitalization" and resulting disruption of cellular calcium regulation. Passive entry of calcium in devitalized cells leads to apatite formation by reacting with cellular phosphorus, this is then followed by calcification of the glutaraldehyde-fixed component. A second mechanism may also occur independently of the collagen, where the elastin fibres in the heart valve are degraded by proteinases as an initial step in deposit formation [Bailey et al., 2003].

Bioprosthetic heart valves are also prone to stress related degeneration. Recently, it has been found that glutaraldehyde does not fix all components of tissue, in particular the glycosaminoglycans and elastin present in the tissues. These components are vulnerable to enzyme and stress related degeneration [Simionescu et al., 2003]. The central spongiosa layer of the porcine heart valve is also vulnerable to embrittlement and eventual tearing [Vyvavahare et al., 1999; Grande-Allen et al., 2003]. During service, the spongiosa become thinner and less flexible. It is found that the composition of glycosaminoglycans, which generate the resilience of the spongiosa, varies with period of service and storage prior to implantation. There is selective leaching of chondroitin-6-sulfate and hyaluronan from the glycosaminoglycans to change their overall composition to mainly chondroitin/dermatan-4-sulfate. This change in composition is consistent with a loss of compressive resistance and visco-elasticity of the spongiosa [Grande-Allen et al., 2003]. The processing of porcine bioprostheses and their subsequent in-service degradation mechanisms are summarized schematically in Figure 5.3

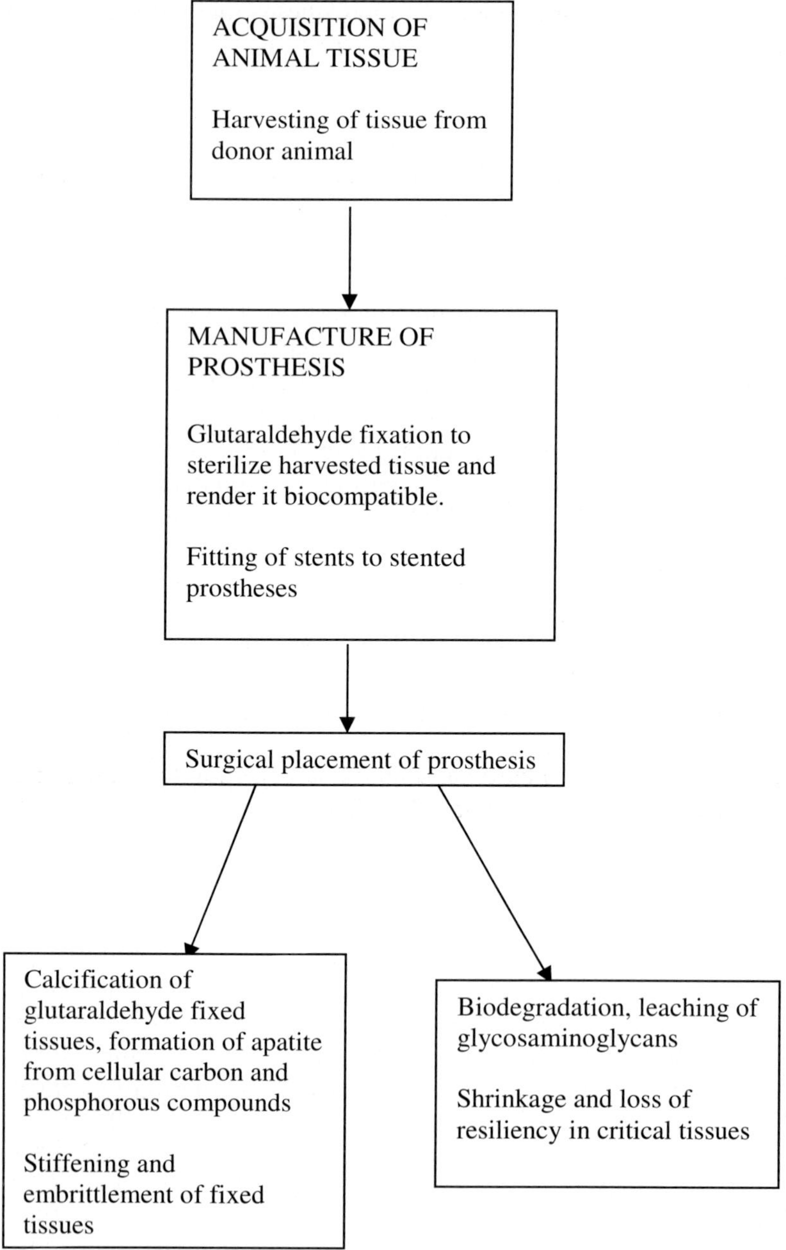

Fig 5.3. Preparation of porcine bioprostheses and events inside body.

To summarize, some of the typical undesirable effects in the patient with artificial valve implantation are listed below.

5.3.1.2   <u>Bioprostheses</u>

Uncertain durability, typically only 10 to 15 years [Grande-Allen et al., 2003]

Reproducible manufacturing is difficult since the prostheses are hand-made from animal tissues of naturally varying characteristics

Calcification and hardening of bioprosthesis after prolonged service

Biodegradation from sustained service inside the human body

Infection risks whether during surgery or from the xenograft itself

5.3.1.3   <u>Mechanical heart valves</u>

Un-natural form and material properties such as elastic modulus

Un-natural flow through the rigid structure of a mechanical valve

Danger of thrombus formation and blood damage due to stagnation areas and high shear stresses within the flow field

Lifelong anti-coagulation treatment necessary for the patient

Noise and Cavitation

Given the problems with using xenografts as sources for heart valves, several new approaches such as new tissue fixation methods, cryopreservation and stentless valves [David, 1998] or even tissue engineered valves are being followed [Steinhoff et al., 2000]. Other substitutes are polymeric valves [Yamagishi et al., 2002], which are currently being developed by several research groups around the world. One approach is to manufacture an artificial valve made of material with properties closely resembling nature tissue. A candidate material is a hydrogel made of polyvinyl alchohol (PVA) [Wan et al., 2002]. Hydrogels are very soft and flexible materials, very different from the rigid metals typically used in artificial heart valves. After a carefully controlled process of freezing and thawing, the PVA hydrogel is found to have mechanical properties such as the stress-relaxation curve very similar to porcine tissue. A flexible stent made of the PVA hydrogel would not suffer from the problems of tearing encountered by rigid metal stents [Wan et al., 2002].

5.3.2 *Environmental and Functional requirements*

Blood is not an inert fluid, instead there is almost some form of reaction between the various constituents of the blood, cells, proteins, dissolved fats etc., and the implanted biomaterial.   Cellular proteins exert a major role during interactions between biomaterials and blood [Vroman, 2003]. When cellular proteins are confined within their cells, several different metabolic systems control the proteins [Vroman, 2003]. If the proteins manage to escape the cells, they will adsorb onto any biomaterial that is present.   Adsorption of proteins, such as immunoglobulins, usually involves distortion of the protein from its normal coiled state. The distortion of immunoglobulins may be sufficient to initiate a larger-scale immune response [Vroman, 2003].   Proteins not only absorb on to artificial surfaces but are also capable of activating leaching of the artificial material into the blood. Serum proteins are capable of binding strongly with metals such as cobalt and titanium to cause very high serum concentrations of these metals [Hallab et al., 2003]. While such elevations in metal concentration are commonly associated with the wear debris around orthopaedic implants, a similar effect cannot be excluded from metal vascular implants.

The contents of the blood are also vulnerable to damage after interaction with artificial materials. A major consideration of any heart valve is the avoidance of blood cell trauma through excessive fluid shear. Erythrocytes (red blood cells) are easily damaged by fluid shear with the possible release of haemoglobin and other metabolites into the serum [Sutera, 1997]. Even if the erythrocytes are not destroyed by shearing (haemolysis), small-scale damage on the cell membrane may occur leading to leakage of cell contents [Ohta et al., 2000]

Stagnant flow regions caused by reverse flow may also cause hyperplasia of blood cells. Prediction of reverse flow, stagnant regions and excessive shear rates is complicated by the fact that blood is a non-Newtonian fluid with high-suspended particle content.

Clotting of blood is unacceptable yet easily provoked by mechanical structures. For instance, the shaft of an artificial heart pump is observed to act as a site for clotting [Akatmatsu]. For this reason, a shaft-less pump with a magnetically suspended impeller is preferred. However, it should be noted that the lower efficiency of magnetic suspension compared to a shaft drive would lead to a higher heat emission for a given flow output. Clotting is manifested in the following ways, formation of a thrombus, formation of a fibrin network over the implant surface and cell adhesion [Iwasaki et al., Swier et al., 1989]. Besides the destructive effects caused by fluid flow in the blood pump, operational factors such as cavitations can lead to hemolysis and destruct system components. Therefore it is important to take these factors into consideration and avoid regions of stagnation, recirculation and low wall shear stress [Tran et al.; Park et al.; Basmadjian; Norris]

The normal human heart beats approximately 38 million times a year which means a mechanical heart valve with a life of 5 years would require to operate for at least 190 million times (without taking into consideration of light exercises performed by the patient). Since the operational environment of heart valve is hostile to artificial materials, it is imperative for the designer to take in to consideration these factors before deciding on the particular material. Blood and extra-cellular fluids are extremely corrosive and can promote various forms of corrosion in metallic materials. On the other hand use of polymeric materials in devices such as vascular catheters or external rings on heart valves may be susceptible to diffusion of mass across these materials by water, oxygen and carbon dioxide. Excessive erosive and cavitation wear may also occur during transport of fluids. A significant factor in the use of prosthetic implants is the inhibition to coagulation. Therefore a balance of anticoagulant properties and procoagulation of prosthetic implant are essential.

5.3.3 *Wear and fracture of heart valves*

Mechanical durability of heart valves depends on the properties of materials used and a material with a good biocompatibility may be inferior when durability is considered. Problems associated with the wear of prosthetic heart valve include generation of rough surfaces, which can enhance thrombosis, induce flow turbulence and expose the sewn ring that encloses the implant. A designer should ideally strike a compromise between biocompatibility and durability with due consideration to toxicity and functional requirements before designing the prostheses. A potential cause of wear in heart valves is cavitation, fluid erosion may also occur for susceptible materials. Cavitation involves bubble formation in regions of liquid flow where the pressure is reduced by either hydrodynamic or hydrostatic effects. Where the cause of bubble formation is hydrodynamic (e.g. downstream flow from an opening), the bubbles periodically form and then collapse. Bubble collapse is destructive to any solid surface since large contact stresses occur whenever the collapsing bubble causes liquid to impact against the solid surface. As a result, fatigue or fracture occurs in the surface material leading to detachment of fragments of surface material [Stachowiak and Batchelor, 2000]. A high velocity of fluid flow also exerts a strong scouring effect on materials, even at the moderate speeds associated with blood flow. It is fortunate that passivated metals such as titanium have very limited solubility in blood, or else erosive wear would be highly significant.

The cavitation causes pit formation on the heart valve surface, the pits may act as sites for crack nucleation in fatigue failure of the heart valve [Chew et al., 2000; Chandran and Aluri, 1997; Bluestein et al., 1994; Hwang, 1998]. Abrasive and erosive wear of valve parts continue to be vital issues during design of mechanical prosthetic valve. The introduction of pyrolytic carbon has been a major advancement in the wear treatment of prosthetic valves. Pyrolytic carbon on pyrolytic carbon has lower wear rates compared to pyrolytic carbon on metals. In some valve designs, a metallic ring reinforces the structurally weak carbon valve housing, in order to avoid deformation of the housing. Deformation of the housing might be associated with jamming of the valve occluders. In some cases titanium is used for the metal frame. Another important problem associated with use of metallic or pyrolytic carbon prostheses is the poor fatigue life, which is still poorly understood. Surface treatments such as ion implantation may improve the fatigue life of metallic implants [Yoganathan] and should be considered when designing heart valves made of pyrolytic carbon and metallic materials. The mechanism of cavitation of biomaterials by the flowing blood is illustrated schematically in Figure 5.4.

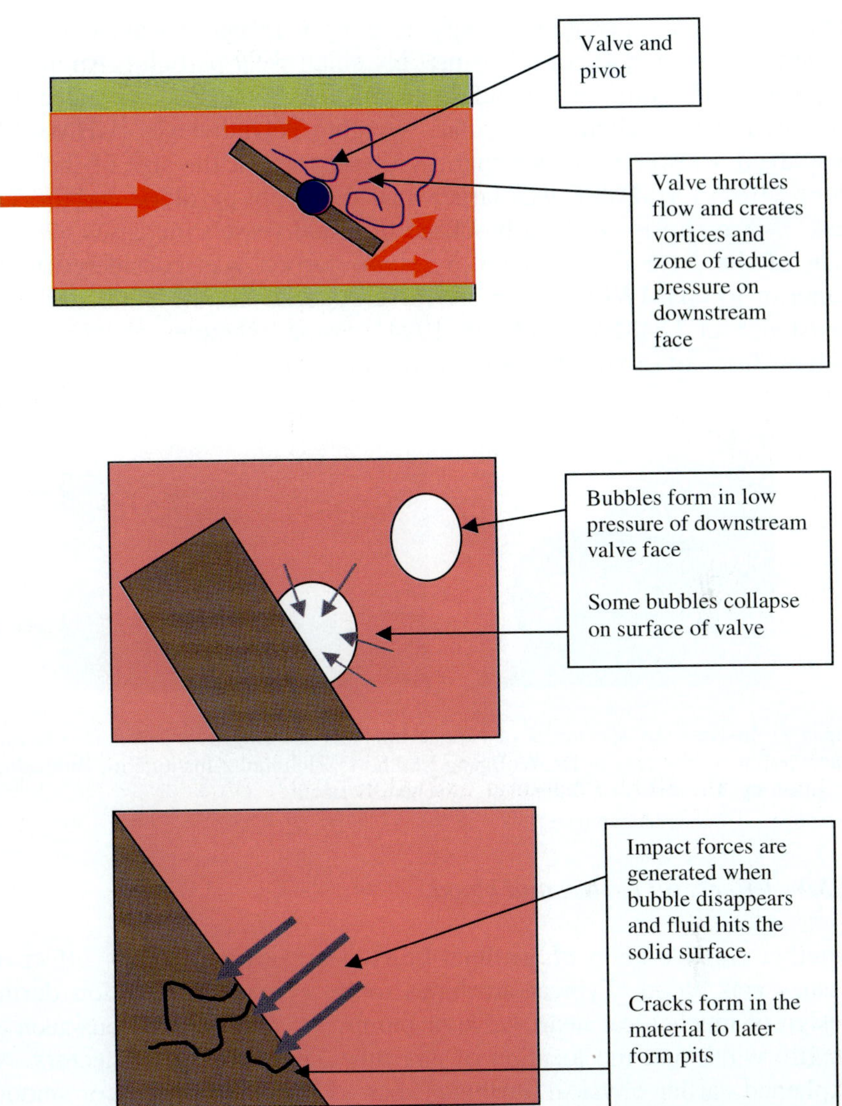

Fig 5.4. Mechanisms of cavitational wear of materials for vascular implants.

The valve material should not only have a good wear resistance, but also have the characteristic of releasing only small wear particles. An in-vitro experimental study of candidate heart valve materials revealed that although Ultra High Molecular Weight Polyethylene (UHMWPE) displayed a lower wear rate than pyrolytic carbon, the size of the wear debris from UHMWPE was larger than that from pyrolytic carbon. The risk of thrombosis or direct blockage of blood vessels increases with the size of the wear debris. Thus pyrolytic carbon was considered to be superior to UHMWPE as a heart valve material despite the better wear resistance of UHMWPE [Teoh, 1994]. Some examples of worn heart valves, from an in-vitro test are shown in Figure 5.5.

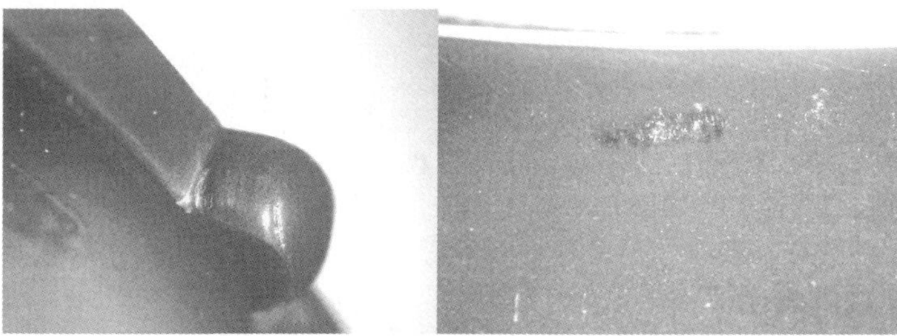

Fig 5.5. In-vitro test specimens of cardiac implants showing wear scars after testing. Photographs by courtesy of Dr. Wolfgang Kerkhoffs, Helmholtz-Institute for Biomedical Engineering, University of Technology, Aachen, Germany.

5.3.4 *Effects on tissues and blood*

Another consideration of artificial heart assist devices is their effect on tissues and blood. Typical attributes to be given consideration during design of mechanical heart valve or pumps are their dimensions such as length, width and the location of any tubes, conduits or connectors. As explained earlier physical attributes such as hard, soft, rough or smooth surfaces and actual shape such as sharp corners or edges that may damage the tissues or organs should be avoided during the design of the artificial heart assist or vascular assist devices. Processes such as wear and fracture of artificial heart devices may lead to one or few of the above circumstances. In addition to this generation of excessive shear stress during flow of blood in blood pumps must be avoided. Wear of mechanical heart valve may result in increase in local shear stress and turbulence in flow. Turbulence fields created by various valve designs and operational consequences can lead to thrombosis and embolism, tissue overgrowth, hemolysis and damage to endothelium adjacent to the valve. Flow induced damage of erythrocytes (red blood cells) is illustrated schematically in Figure 5.6.

Laminar flow shear stresses can also lead to blood cell damage if the shear stresses are comparable to those found in turbulent flow. Moreover the shear induced platelet damage is cumulative as the combination of shear magnitude and time of exposure may not induce platelet aggregation while accumulated damage as a result of multiple journeys through the artificial valve may be sufficient to cause thrombosis and subsequent embolization. Artificial heart assist devices increase the chances of blood cell damage in the event of high turbulent shear stress because of the presence of surfaces composed of alien materials. In addition to this flow stagnation and/or flow separation that occur adjacent to the valve either due to the design or due to the operational consequences (wear) could promote deposition of damaged blood elements and thrombus formation. Thus a significant disadvantage of mechanical valves is the need for continuous anti coagulation therapy to avoid thrombosis and thrombo-embolic complications. Careful anti coagulation therapy is required in order to avoid consequential bleeding problems.

5.4 Stents for cardiac blood vessels

Stents have gained prominence in the treatment of cardio vascular diseases. Most common materials used are stainless steel in current practice though titanium and titanium alloys (Ni Ti) are also being used. The function intended is to dilate and keep narrowed blood vessels open. They are usually mounted on balloon catheters or folded inside special delivery catheters. They are introduced into the vascular systems by puncturing and guided to specific locations using X rays. On reaching the desired location the balloon is inflated and the stent expands to a predetermined size. During placement of stents there are inevitable damages to the blood vessel wall, which leads to the risk of thrombotic occlusion due to the presence of stent material, which is a foreign body. One of the significant problems associated with titanium alloys stents is their poor radio opacity compared to stainless steel.

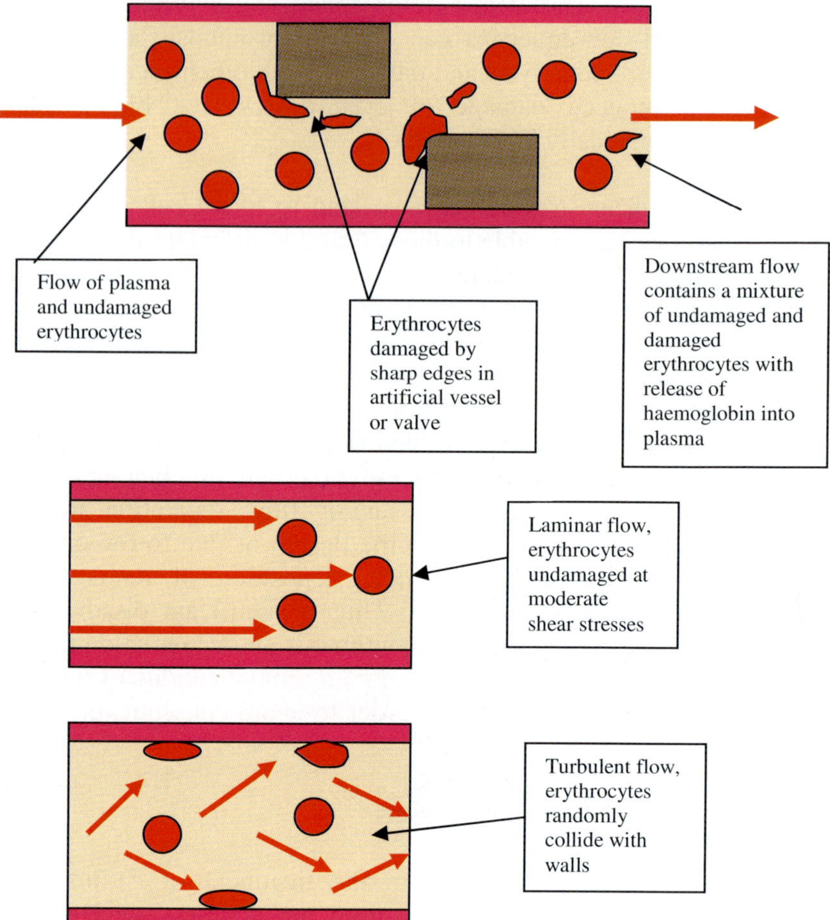

Fig 5.6. Flow induced haemolysis or damage to erythrocytes.

A major problem with the use of stents is the physical structure involving corrugation, kinks and steps, which generate pockets of abnormal blood flow. Recirculating blood flow and prolonged residence of blood at specific sites are associated with undesirable changes in the blood such as thrombosis and myointimal hyperplasia (MIH, see below) [Chong, How and Harris].

An implanted stent may not always remain open for blood flow, instead cellular growth inside the stent can cause blockage of the stent. Subsequent blockage of the stent after implantation is known as restenosis. Restenosis may not only be caused by clotting and cell growth, but also by an allergic response [Koster et al., 2000]. The metal alloys used to make stents contain nickel and molybdenum. Nickel is known to provoke an allergic response in 10% of women and 1-2% of men, while the allergic potential of molybdenum has not yet been quantified [Keane, 2001]. Restenosis of a stent is shown schematically in Figure 5.7.

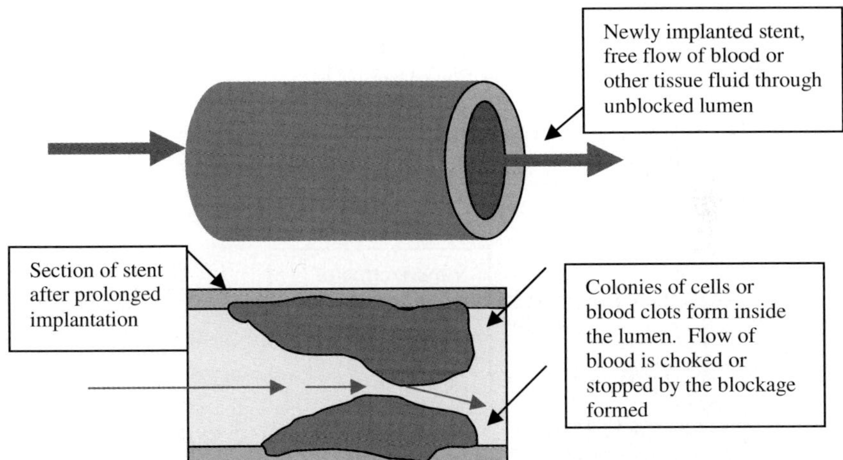

Fig 5.7. Mechanism of restenosis in a stent.

New designs of stents to overcome the problems of stenosis and thrombosis are continually being developed. For instance, an elastomeric (rubbery) film with micro-pored covering has been developed to prevent restenosis [Nakayama et al., 2003]. The elastomeric film is made of a base layer of polyurethane with a blood-compatible inner layer of photo-reactive gelatin and heparin. Heparin is an anti-clotting agent and the gelatin was cured (hardened or solidified by development of cross-linked chemical bonds) by exposure to Ultra-Violet light (UV). The pores in the polyurethane were formed by ablation using pulsed radiation from an excimer laser. The excimer laser is a pulsed UV laser with a very high photo-intensity. Under this intense UV, the chemical bonds of atoms and molecules beneath the irradiated surface are cut to release the molecules. The excimer laser is different from the carbon dioxide laser, which induces intense localized heating. Ablation means the vaporization of material when intense energy is applied. The purpose of the micro-pores, average diameter 30 micrometres and average spacing 125 micrometres is to suppress cellular growth (as in restenosis)[Nakayama et al., 2003]. The process of forming micro-pores and the resultant surface is shown schematically in Figure 5.8.

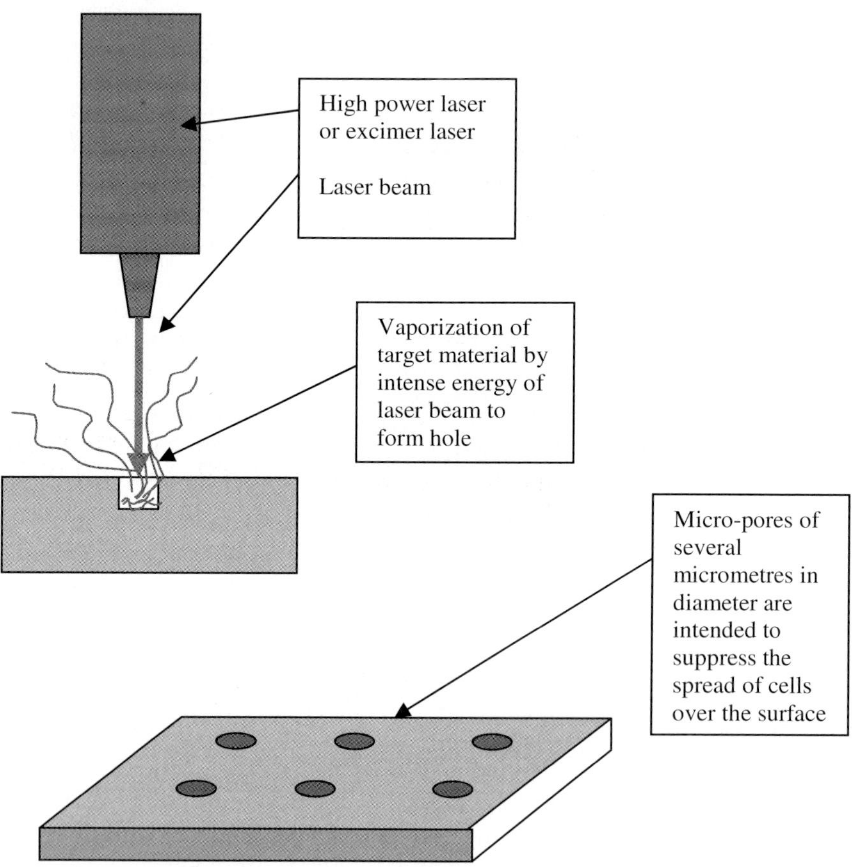

Fig 5.8. Micro-pore formation by ablation and the control of restenosis. [Nakayama et al., 2003].

In a related research project, a smaller diameter artificial graft was designed with comparable mechanical stiffness to natural arteries [Sonoda et al., 2003]. Efficient blood flow (maximum flow rate for minimum pumping power) is enhanced by the property of arteries to expand and contract with variation in flow output from the heart [Kinley and Marble, 1980]. A double tube coaxial design of artificial graft was developed and found to maintain a mechanical compliance similar to natural arteries [Sonoda et al., 2003].

There are several types of stent coatings, not just the gelatin-heparin coating described above. A phosphoryl-choline based polymer coating was found to be still intact after 6 months implantation in a human patient [Lewis et al., 2002].   The diameter of the blood vessel is of critical importance to the design of vascular implants.   Implants with less than 6 mm diameter suffer from the problem ensuring that an endothelium can form inside the lumen (interior space) of the graft and some methods involving proprietary materials have been proposed [Carnagey et al., 2003].

5.5 Implantation of pacemakers

Pacemakers were originally cased in Epoxy resins or silicon rubber. Though this worked well clinically, it did produce undesirable foreign body reactions, which could have led to infections [Naegeli and Bertel, 2003; Engelstein, 2003]. Titanium has been used as replacement material for shielding and has proven to work well with lower incidents of fluid accumulation and infection. Common complications associated with the implantation of pacemakers include bleeding, infection, lead dislodgement and lead or pacemaker problem during surgery. Venous access is the most frequent cause of significant complications during implantation of the pacemaker. Pneumothorax, hemothorax, air embolism, and perforation of a central vein or the heart can be caused by the venous access.

5.6 Vascular implants

Arteries remote from the heart in locations such as the limbs are prone to blockage by plaques and clots. The artery may be treated by creating a diversion to the blocked section of the artery. The diversion can be constructed from a section of vein taken from the patient's body or from an artificial material such as Polytetrafluoroethylene (PTFE) tubing. A major problem with an arterial prosthesis (*i.e.,* the PTFE tubing), is poor performance when the diversion is sited below the knee [How et al., 2000]. A problem known as Myointimal Hyperplasia (MIH) (abnormal multiplication or increase in number of cells in a normal arrangement in a tissue) occurs at the junction of the graft with the original blood vessel. The occurrence of MIH leads to tissue in-growth, which chokes the flow of blood [Nakayama et al., 2003]. A further effect of MIH is to cause thrombosis (formation of blood clot), which blocks the arterial prosthesis. MIH is associated with low wall shear stress in the blood flow through the graft; it appears that a strong sweeping action is required to maintain functionality of the blood vessel. Low wall shear stress and MIH are usually sited close to the point where the flow is diverted from the original artery and are suppressed by fitting a chamber to the site of flow diversion. This is shown in Figure 5.9.

Polyurethane is widely used for small diameter vascular prostheses because of its favourable mechanical properties and high level of biocompatibility. The viscoelasticity of polyurethane can be adjusted so that the mechanical compliance of the prosthesis is closely similar to that of the natural artery [Chong et al., 2000]. The vascular prosthesis is formed from electro statically spun fibers of medical-grade polyurethane (diameter approximately 1 - 2 micrometers). It is found that polyurethane is able to support an adhering layer of endothelial and smooth muscle cells [Chong et al., 2000].

5.7 Neural implants

Nerve guidance conduits are currently being developed for use in surgical repair of nerve injury. High levels of biocompatibility and biodegradability are critical for the avoidance of damage to sensitive neural tissues. A biodegradable implant enables omission of the surgical removal of the nerve conduit. If the implant neither self-destructs nor is removed, the patient may suffer pain from nerve compression. A major consideration in biodegradability, apart from the rate of degradation, is the biocompatiblity of the degradation products. Polyphosphate ester has been proposed as a material because its decomposition products are phosphate, alcohol and diol, which are believed to be not harmful to tissues adjacent to the nerve conduit [Wang et al., 2000]. Polyphosphate is decomposed by hydrolysis in the presence of nucleophiles such as hydroxyl ions. It was observed that degradation *in vivo* proceeded slower than under comparable conditions *in vitro*. The slower rate *in vivo* may be due to shielding of hydroxyl ions by fibrous tissue formed around the implant [Wang et al., 2000].

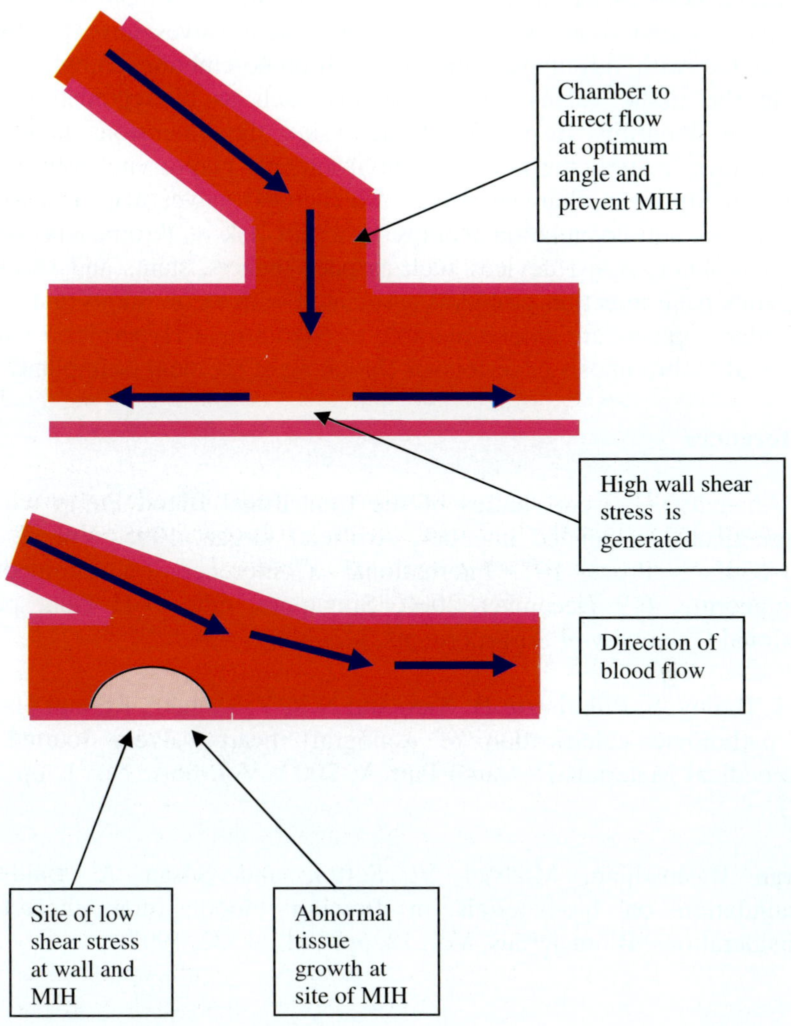

Fig 5.9. Flow geometry, wall shear stress and thrombosis risk in arterial prostheses.

Neural implants are a recent development and the information available on basic service characteristics such as long-term durability remains very limited. With progress in research and clinical testing, it is expected that more information will become available in the future.

5.8 Summary

Artificial heart assist valves can be classified into two main categories; mechanical and tissue valves. The mechanical valves have problems associated with thrombosis and other thrombo-embolic complications while the tissue valves have problems such as biodegradation and uncertain durability. Besides the basic design, the dimensions, mass and the surface features the operating environments play a vital role in the functionality of mechanical valves. Mechanical valves also necessitate continuous anti-coagulation therapy to avoid risk of thrombosis. Heart and circulatory assist devices such as pace makers, stents and vascular implants have infection problems associated with them. Stents and other vascular implants are also vulnerable to Myointimal Hyperplasia which can lead to thrombosis or restenosis (blocking of the stent or implant).

References

T. Akamatsu, Present studies of the Centrifugal Blood Pump with a Magnetically suspended impeller, Artificial Organ, 1995, Vol. 7, pp. 631-634. , Proc. 10th International Conference on Biomedical Engineering, 6-9 December 2000, Singapore, edit. JCH Goh, publ. National University of Singapore, pp. 343-344.

M.T. Bailey, S. Pillarisetti, H. Xiao and N.R. Vyavahare, Role of elastin in pathologic calcification of xenograft heart valves, Journal of Biomedical Materials Research Part A, 2003, Vol. 66A, No. 1, pp. 93-102.

Diran Basmadjian, Michael V. Sefton and Susan A. Baldwin, Coagulation on biomaterials in flowing blood: some theoretical considerations. Biomaterials, Vol. 18, pp. 1511-1522, 1997.

D. Bluestein, S. Einav and N.H.C. Hwang, A squeeze flow phenomenon at the closing of a Bileaflet Mechanical Heart Vale Prosthesis, Journal of Biomechanics, 1994, Vol. 27, No. 11, pp. 1369-1378.

J. Carnagey, D. Hern-Anderson, J. Ranieri and C.E. Schmidt, Rapid endothelialization of PhotoFix natural biomaterial vascular grafts, Journal of Biomedical Materials Research, 2003, Vol. 65B, No. 1, pp. 171-179.

K.B. Chandran and Aluri, Mechanical Valve closing dynamics, relationship between velocity of closing, pressure transients and cavitation initiation, Journal of Biomechanical Engineering, 1997, Vol. 25, pp. 926-938.

W. Chen, F.J. Schoey, R.J. Levy, Mechanisms of efficacy of 2-amino oleic acid for the inhibition of calcification of glutaraldehyde-pretreated porcine bioprosthetic heart valves, 1994, Circulation, Vol. 90, pp. 323-329.

Y.T. Chew, H.T. Low and Sun Yuqing, A numerical study of closing dynamics and cavitation in mechanical heart valves, Proc. 10th International Conference on Biomedical Engineering, 6-9 December 2000, Singapore, edit. JCH Goh, publ. National University of Singapore, pp. 351-352.

C.K. Chong, T.V. How and P.L. Harris, Endografting of aortic aneurysms, in vitro applications, clinical implications, Proc. 10th International Conference on Biomedical Engineering, 6-9 December 2000, Singapore, edit. JCH Goh, publ. National University of Singapore, pp. 189-190.

Shayne Cox Gad, Safety Evaluation of Medical Devices, 2nd Edition,2002, Marcel Dekker Inc., pp. 477-504.

Erica D. Engelstein, Prevention and Management of Chronic Heart Failure with Electrical Therapy, Proceedings of Symposium on From Prevention to Management of Chronic Heart Failure, The American Journal of Cardiology, 2003, Vol. 91 (9A) May 8, 2003, pp. 62F-73F.

K.J. Grande-Allen, W.J. Mako, A. Calabro, Y. Shi, N.B. Ratliff and I. Vesely, Loss of chondroitin 6-sulfate and hyaluronan from failed porcine bioprosthetic valves, Journal of Biomedical Materials Research Part A, 2003, No. 2, pp. 251-259.

H. Haferkampf, T. Fabian, K. Kaese, M. Niemeyer, K. Philipp, B. Heublein and R. Rohde, Magnesium as a degradable metallic biomaterial, Proc. 10th International Conference on Biomedical Engineering, 6-9th December 2000, Singapore, edit. JCH Goh, publ. National University of Singapore, pp. 509-510.

N.H.C. Hwang, Cavitation potential of pyrolytic carbon heart valve prostheses, a review and current status, The Journal of Heart Valve Disease, 1998, Vol. 7, pp. 140-150.

K.Iwasaki, M. Umezu, K. Imachi, K. Iijima, M. Morita and C.X. Ye, In-vitro performance tests of a newly-developed bileaflet polymer valve,

F.M. Keane, S.D. Morris, H.R. Smith, R.J.G. Rycroft, Allergy in coronary in-stent restenosis, The Lancet, 2001, Vol. 357, No. 9263, 14 April 2001.
http://www.thelancet.com/journal/vol357/iss9263/full/llan.357.9263.corr espondence.15856.1

C.E. Kinley and A.E. Marble, Compliance: a continuing problem with vascular grafts, 1980, Journal of Cardiovascular Surgery, Vol. 21, pp. 163-170.

R. Koster, D. Vieluf, M.Kiehn, M. Sommerauer, J. Kahler, S. Baldus, T. Meinertz and C.W. Hamm, Nickel and molybdenum contact allergies in patients with coronary in-stent restenosis, The Lancet, 2000, Vol. 356, pp. 1895-1897.

N.J. Hallab, A. Skipor and J.J. Jacobs, Interfacial kinetics of titanium- and cobalt-based implant alloys in human serum: Metal release and biofilm formation, Journal of Biomedical Materials Research, Part A, 2003, Vol. 65A, No. 3, pp. 311-318.

T.V. How, C. S. Rowe, G.L. Gilling-Smith and P.L. Harris, Improving wall shear stress distribution in lower limb arterial bypass, Proc. 10th International Conference on Biomedical Engineering, 6-9 December 2000, Singapore, edit. JCH Goh, publ. National University of Singapore, pp.401-402.

A.L. Lewis, J. D. Furze, S. Small, J.D. Robertson, B.J. Higgins, S. Taylor and D.R. Ricci, Long-term stability of a coronary stent coating post-implantation, Journal of Biomedical Materials Research, 2002, Vol. 63, No. 6, pp. 699-705.

Barbara Naegeli and Osmund Bertel, No body is perfect—a pacemaker dysfunction, International Journal of cardiology, Article in Press.

Y. Nakayama, S. Nishi, H. Ueda-Ishibashi and T. Matsuda, Fabrication of micropored elastomeric film-covered stents and acute-phase performances, Journal of Biomedical Materials Research, Part A, 2003, Vol. 64A, No. 1, pp. 52-61.

Lucy A. Norris, Blood Coagulation, Best Practice & Research Clinical Obstetrics & Gynaecology, Vol. 17, No. 3, pp. 369–383, 2003.

Christian Olin, Titanium in Cardiac & Cardiovascular Applications, Titanium in Medicine, Ed. D M. Brunette, P.Tengvall, M.Textor, P.Thomsen, Springer Verlag Publications, 2001, pp. 889-908.

Y. Ohta, H. Okamoto, F. Saito and T. Okuda, Atomic force microscopic visualization of sheared erythrocytes: effect of periodic flow on the surface roughness, Proc. 10th International Conference on Biomedical Engineering, 6-9 December 2000, Singapore, edit. JCH Goh, publ. National University of Singapore, pp. 83-84.

K.D. Park, Y.H. Kim, W.K. Lee, Novel Modification method of bioprosthetic tissue for improved calcification resistance, Biomaterials Engineering and Devices: Human Applications, Vol. 1: Fundamentals and Vascular and Carrier applications, Ed. Donald L.Wise, Debra J. Trantolo, Kai-Uwe Lewandrowski, Joseph D. Gresser, Mario V. Cattaneo and Michael J. Yaszemski, 2000, publ. Humana Press, Totowa, New Jersey, USA, pp. 49-56.

H.R. Pilcher, Human arteries grown from scratch, Nature Science Updates, 6th June 2003,
http://www.nature.com/nsu/030602/030602-15.html

Gerson Rosenverg, Artificial heart and circulatory assist devices, the biomedical engineering hand book 2nd edition, vol. 2, Ed. Joseph D. Bronzino CRC & IEEE Press, pp. 126/1-126/8.

Christine E. Schmidt and Jennie M. Baier, Acellular vascular tissues: natural biomaterials for tissue repair and tissue engineering, Biomaterials, 2000, Vol. 21, pp. 2215-2231.

H. Sonoda, K. Takamizawa, Y. Nakayama, H. Yasui and T. Matsuda, Coaxial double-tubular compliant arterial graft prosthesis: Time-dependent morphogenesis and compliance changes after implantation, Journal of Biomedical Materials Research Part A, 2003, Vol. 65A, No. 2, pp. 170-181.

G.W. Stachowiak and A.W. Batchelor, Engineering Tribology, 2nd edition, publ. Butterworth-Heinemann, 2001, Boston, USA.

S.P. Sutera, Flow-induced trauma to blood cells, Circulation Research, 1977, Vol. 41, No. 1, pp. 2-8.

P. Swier, W.J. Bos, S.F. Mohammad, D.B. Olsen and W.J. Kolff, An in-vitro test model to study the performance and thrombogenecity of cardiovascular devices, Transactions ASAIO, 1989, Vol. 35, pp. 683-687.

Teoh, Swee Hin, Private seminar, National University of Singapore, 1994.

H.S. Trang, M.M. Puc, F.A. Chrzanowski, C.W. Hewitt, D.B. Soll, B. Sing, N. Kumar, S. Marra and V. Simonetti, Surface Modifications of Mechanical Heart Valves; Effects on Thrombogenicity, Biomaterials Engineering and Devices: Human Applications, Vol. 1: Fundamentals and Vascular and Carrier applications, Ed. Donald L.Wise, Debra J. Trantolo, Kai-Uwe Lewandrowski, Joseph D. Gresser, Mario V. Cattaneo and Michael J. Yaszemski, 2000, publ. Humana Press, Totowa, New Jersey, USA, pp. 137-144.

L. Vroman, Perspectives on blood/materials interactions, Journal of Biomedical Materials Research, Part A, 2003, Vol. 65A, No. 2, page 125.

W.K. Wan, G. Campbell, Z.F. Zhang, A.J. Hui and D.R. Boughner, Optimizing the tensile properties of polyvinyl alcohol hydrogel for the construction of a bioprosthetic heart valve stent, Journal of Biomedical Materials Research, 2002, Vol. 63, No. 6, pp. 854-861.

S. Wang, A.C.A. Wan, H.-Q. Mao, H. Yu and K.W. Leong, Biodegradable poly(phospoester) tubes promotes peripheral nerve regeneration, Proc. 10th International Conference on Biomedical Engineering, 6-9 December 2000, Singapore, edit. JCH Goh, publ. National University of Singapore, pp. 124-125.

C.-Y. Lee, N. Vyavahare, R. Zand, H. Kruth, F.J. Schoen, R. Bianco and R.J. Levy, Inhibition of aortic wall calcification in bioprosthetic heart valves by ethanol pretreatment: Biochemical and biophysical mechanisms, Journal of Biomedical Materials Research, 1998, Vol. 42, No. 1, 1998, pp. 30-37.

Ajit. P.Yoganathan, Cardiac Valve Prostheses, The biomedical engineering hand book 2nd edition, vol. 2, Ed. Joseph D. Bronzino CRC & IEEE Press, pp. 127/1-127/23.

Chapter 6

Dental Implants

6.1 Introduction

Teeth of most modern mammal species including humans are highly developed structures where opposing teeth are closely interlocked during chewing and biting. A precise interlock between teeth is necessary for the food to be efficiently cut and shredded by the teeth. Closely interlocking teeth are termed 'tribosphenic' [Liu et al., 2001, Shackleton, 2001] and are fundamentally more advanced than the teeth of earlier mammals, which merely sliced past each other during chewing. The tribosphenic quality of teeth is so important that modern mammalian teeth are believed to have evolved from two separate and independent sources [Liu et al., 2001]. The structure of human teeth is also remarkable, since human teeth must resist fracture despite the millions of chewing movements and other tooth contacts that occur in a lifetime. It has been observed that the junction between the surface layer of enamel and the inner layer of dentine is sufficiently tough to deflect or stop most cracks that form on the enamel from propagating into the dentin [Dong and Ruse, 2003]. The mechanical properties of the dentin-enamel interface are found to be critical for crack suppression. Human saliva is also critical for the protection of natural teeth from wear since it acts as a lubricant and coolant during chewing and rapid wear of teeth will occur when salivation is disrupted [Li and Zhou, 2002]. Despite such evolutionary sophistications, tooth loss is common during a human lifetime and dental implants may be required to ensure effective chewing of food.

Besides the tooth loss, corrective measures to set the alignment of the upper jaw and dentures are often required in patient's requiring special needs. The implant materials used in dentistry can be broadly classified as permanent and temporary based on their applications. It can also be classified as synthetic or natural materials. Some of the natural materials include bone grafts which are either autografts or the xenografts. The development of new dental implants or related treatment systems is the focus of much current interest. A recent development is the formulation of a new cement containing calcium phosphate and other minerals, which suppresses the growth of bacterial colonies around the fixture sites of dental braces [Skrtic et al., 2003]. Bacterial colonies usually flourish around such fixture sites because they are difficult to reach with a cleaning brush.

In the dental context, an implant refers only to a prosthetic device made of an *alloplastic* (synthetic) material that is placed (implanted) either below the mucosal layer or the periosteal layer of the oral tissues or deeper within the bone. The purpose of the implant is to provide a secure base or support for a permanently attached or removable prosthesis, such as an artificial tooth crown [Glossary of Prosthodontic Terms].   Other artificial materials placed within dental tissues are referred to as biomaterials.

6.2 Origins of dental decay and tooth loss

Dental decay, known as caries, is the result of a bacterial infection of the tooth surfaces. When foods, especially sugars, are consumed, bacteria present on the teeth surfaces convert the food ingredients to organic acids. Teeth are covered by plaque, which is a thin layer of bacteria, human cells and particulate matter. The organic acids generated by bacteria corrode the enamel coating of the teeth, since the enamel contains calcium phosphate. This process of corrosive damage to the enamel is known as demineralization. Once the enamel is perforated by acidic corrosion, the soft tissues within the tooth become vulnerable to further infection by bacteria. Caries is found in animals as well as humans, with rats being widely used as experimental models of humans for caries studies.

Studies on rats kept in sterile conditions have shown that the mere consumption of sugars is not sufficient to cause caries, which is directly related to the presence of mouth bacteria. Bacteria from the relatively common streptococcus genus, *streptococcus mutans*, is found to be closely associated with the occurrence of caries in humans [Macpherson et al., 1990]. Bacteria and their waste products may not entirely control caries, there is evidence that components of human saliva may also contribute to caries [Gabrovsek (2), 1997]. The human saliva contains leukocytes that release enzymes, which only function effectively in acidic conditions. These hydrolytic enzymes decompose sugars, fats and proteins as part of the attack response by leukocytes to foreign cellular matter. The enzymes are non-discriminating so they can also attack gum tissue and enamel.

There is evidence of inherited (genetic) predisposition to caries [Gabrovsek (4), 1997] and a gender bias where females are more prone to caries [Gabrovsek (3), 1997].   It is unclear whether the controlling factors in gender bias are physiological or cultural.

Caries and other oral infections are not the only cause of tooth loss. Pathological conditions such as high blood pressure may lead to blood vessel failure in the root of the tooth and accidents, resulting in breakage of a tooth, can necessitate use of artificial materials or implants to restore functionality. Even when the teeth themselves are healthy and undamaged, orthodontic correction is often performed in patients to improve the facial appearance or to realign the upper and lower jaw. Failure to align the jaws can lead to entrapment of food particles within the gaps in the crowded teeth followed by tooth decay due to bacterial action [The Hindu, 2003], [Diane et.al.,2001].

6.3 Materials for dental implants

The implants used in dentistry can be broadly classified into four main categories depending on the type of implant, which are oral implants, prosthodontics, orthodontics and endodontics.

6.3.1 *Oral implants*

Subperiosteal (this means below the periosteum), transosteal and endosseous implants fall under the category of oral implants.

Subperiosteal implants are custom made framework, which rests on the bone surface beneath the muco-periosteum while the transosteal implants are those which are placed in the frontal lower jaw. The muco-periosteum consists of a mucosa (connective tissue layer covered by a layer of mucus) on the exterior (i.e., the surface contacting saliva and food) and a periosteum (thin cellular layer that facilitates bone growth) contacting the bone. Bone plates and transmandibular implants can also be fitted to the frontal lower jaw. In current dental practice, these kinds of implants are almost obsolete. Endossous implants are those that can be placed in the jaws through a mucoperiosteal incision. These are the most commonly used implants, which can be categorized as fixators. Fixators come in many forms such as pins, needles, blades, discs and root formed analogues such as screws, cylinders, hollow implants and various other forms.

6.3.2 *Bone graft materials*

Alveolar bone loss is one of the typical problems associated with tooth loss. The alveolar bone lies adjacent to the teeth and provides the essential structural support for the teeth. The implants used in dentistry without alveolar ridge augmentation often fail or generate a poor aesthetic appearance. In order to have a successful implant alveolar ridge augmentation, a suitable bone graft material is necessary. These bone graft materials can be classified into four different categories namely autografts, allografts, xenografts and alloplasts. In autografts, the bone cells are donated by the patient from e.g., the hip. The allograft is a bone donated by a different member of the same species (human source other than the patient). Xenografts are mineralized bone matrix from a different species while the alloplasts are the synthetic bone materials. Autografts form the best solution followed by allografts and xenografts as the surrounding tissue is more likely to identify the implanted bone graft materials as a compatible counterpart. One of the potential problems with the autografts is morbidity (failure to heal) at the site where the bone cells were taken, thus limiting its use. Allografts often suffer from immunorejection or foreign object rejection reactions by the surrounding tissue. Xenografts suffer from immunorejections and other problems occurring in autografts and allografts, they are also costly. A potential solution to these reported problems would be the use of alloplasts (synthetic bone materials). Biomedical engineers working on dental materials would be more interested in the development and use of alloplasts. These include resorbable and non resorbable materials. Resorbable materials are decomposed and dispersed by the various metabolic and cellular processes occurring within tissues. Non-resorbable materials are intended to remain intact for an indefinite period of time. Tricalcium phosphate, hydroxy appatite (HA) and bioactive glass constitute the resorbable alloplasts while polymers, ceramic HA are the non-resorbable alloplasts. The main advantages of these alloplasts are their availability, their acceptance by the patient, osteo-conductivity and biocompatibility.

The dental implants can be broadly divided into subperiosteal and endosteal categories. Most common sub-periosteal implant is the Co-Cr-Mo alloy while titanium or titanium alloys are used in endosteal implants.

6.4 Materials for dental fixators

One of the major developments in restorative dentistry is the use of materials or alloys. The anchorage between a non biological component and the surrounding hard or soft tissue is facilitated by the use of a non biological anchoring component. These are known as dental fixators which undergo *osseo-integration* with the surrounding tissue. Osseo-integration involves regrowth of bone cells after implantation to form a close bond with the implant or dental biomaterial. Dental fixators are a rapidly developing technology for restorative dentistry. Lost teeth can now be replaced by a porcelain tooth that is secured to the jaw by a fixator. The fixator is usually made of titanium alloy, which is non-toxic and biocompatible. The fixator is divided into a lower section, which is designed to adhere to the jaw bone and an upper threaded portion to secure the artificial tooth. Surgery involves the removal of residual tooth tissue and the preparation of space for a cylindrical or plate shaped fixator. The fixator is then inserted in the jaw and the gum tissue stitched in place. The fixator is then allowed to bond with the bone by the process known as *osseointegration* that lasts several weeks. Once the bond between bone and fixator is sufficiently strong, the artificial tooth can be fitted to the fixator. The patient then uses the tooth in the same manner as a natural tooth, maintaining dental hygiene by brushing and flossing. The concept of a dental fixator and separate dental crown is shown schematically in Figure 6.1, together with the location of the muco-periosteum and the alveolar ridge.

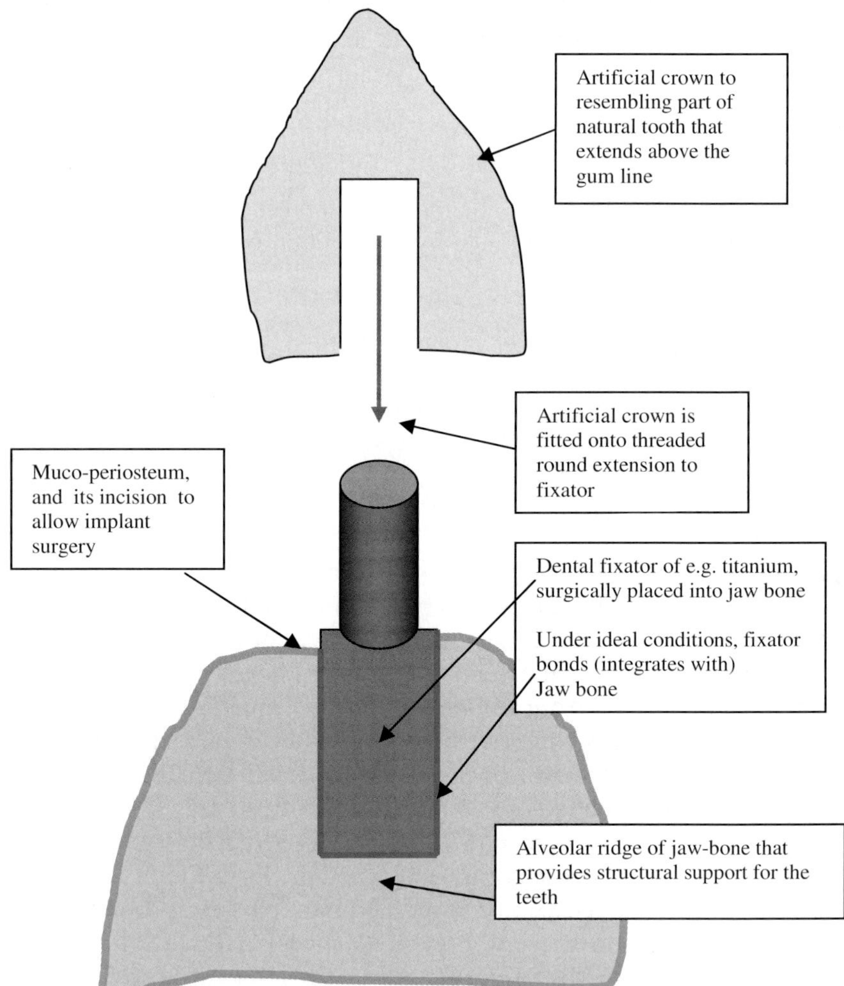

Fig 6.1. Dental fixator and attached dental crown.

There are various candidate materials for substituting deranged structure
(unhealthy or deformed bone and gums), which include Vitallium, pure
titanium and its alloys, PMMA (Poly-Methyl-Methacrylate) and hydroxy
apatite. Of these 'Vitallium™', which is basically Cobalt, Chromium
and Molybdenum alloy, is mainly used in subperiosteal implants, which
are normally fabricated by lost-wax casting. Subperiosteal implants are

mainly used in edentulous regions where endosseous implants cannot be used because of the resorption of the bone. Endosteal implants only require 10 mm depth of bone and subperiosteal implants are rarely used today. Moreover, there are additional problems associated with subperiosteal implants including possible infection and further resorption of bone. Endosteal implants are placed within the bone. Secondary procedures are carried out once the primary wound heals to connect the prosthetic teeth. Endosseous implants can be either in plate form or in root form. Titanium and its alloys are used in endosteal implants. Osseo-integration of Titanium or Titanium alloy implants is normally achieved by direct bone implant contact due to the bio-inert surface layer of Titanium oxide (as discussed in Chapter 3). One of the recent developments is the use of a HA coating on the exterior of titanium endosteal implants to provide a bio-active surface. A bio-active surface promotes bone regrowth (as discussed in Chapter 4).

Titanium has been found to be not only corrosion resistant and strong but is also well tolerated by the body, i.e. it is biocompatible. A study of titanium and various titanium alloys, where the activation of osteoblast-like cells on discs of metal was measured, revealed that commercially pure titanium generated the most activation or stimulation of the cells [Spyrou et al., 2002]. Activation of osteoblasts (bone synthesizing cells) is vital for bone regrowth around the implant. A titanium-vanadium-aluminium alloy used in prosthesis construction caused the least cellular activation. The presence of aluminium and vanadium in this alloy may be the reason for the subdued cellular activity. The cytotoxicity of Vanadium is higher than other metals and has been found to delay the healing process by reduced cellular activation.

While titanium alloys have been found largely by accident to possess a excellent degree of biocompatibility enabling vigorous bone regrowth around a fixator, better biocompatibility may be achieved with a coating on the titanium alloy. One type of coating is based on calcium hydroxyapatite, which is considered to be osteoconductive (promotes bone regrowth inside the coating). Calcium hydroxyapatite is not ideal as a coating material, being comparatively soft and brittle (as discussed in Chapter 4). A 5-year follow-up study revealed no significant difference in the failure rate of implants coated with hydroxyapatite and with titanium [Mau et al. 2002]. Other more conventional coatings, known for wear resistance (resists scratching by the surgeons tools and the bone) have also been considered. Titanium nitride coatings, which is extremely hard and is used to enhance cutting tools, is shown to promote more vigorous attachment and growth by fibroblasts than a plain titanium metal surface [Groessner-Schreiber et al. 2003]. Fibroblasts are the cells, which synthesize the collagens, reticular and elastic fibres, glycosaminoglycans and glycoproteins that form the extracellular matrices of connective tissues. If the fibroblasts can thrive on the surface of the implant, then the chances of tissue re-growth should improve. However, it should be noted that fibrous connective tissue formation around a dental implant is considered undesirable because of the lack of real bonding. Useful bonding occurs when the bone contacts the implant directly without an intervening layer of fibrous connective tissue.

HA coatings and Titanium based implants and fixators have gained prominence because the induced bio-activity, which means successful bone regrowth. Studies have also indicated that HA coated implants show better bone implant contact over uncoated Ti based implant. The level of bone implant bonding achieved with HA coating is beyond Branemark Osseointegration. Despite the advantages of HA coating there are reports of kidney failures and possibility of resorption of the HA surface over a period of time. Potential soft tissue complications also arise if the HA coating becomes exposed to infection. Another problem with HA coating in the case of sub-periosteal implants is the obstruction to forming suspensory tissue slings, which are the primary support mechanism of subperiosteal implants.

6.4.1 *Prosthodontic materials and implants*

Fixed and removable protheses such as dentures belong to this category of implants and dental materials. Artificial teeth made for aesthetic reasons and soft tissue analogues can be similarly classified as prosthodontic materials. Dental restorative materials form a typical prosthodontic application. Titanium is considered as an alternative to noble alloys such as gold dental alloys owing to its high bio-compatibility and non-allergenic nature in combination with relatively low cost.

6.5 Dental restorative materials

Prosthodontic material can be divided into two basic categories, restorative material for correction of dental decay/fissures and artificial teeth to replace lost teeth. For the fillers, the traditional amalgam is being progressively replaced by polymer resins and glass ionomer cements. Dental amalgams were used for filling over 100 years and contain a mixture of mercury and silver. The amalgam solidifies when the inter-metallic compounds form and interlock. Amalgam is easily applied and more durable than other fillers but has the disadvantage of containing mercury, which is highly toxic. New metal alloys for dental amalgams have been developed where toxic metals are excluded and corrosion resistance is enhanced. An example is an alloy, 50% Silver, 30% Tin and 20% Copper, which is processed as a powder [Gem alloy]. A traditional but expensive material is gold, which is alloyed with metals such as silver and palladium for strength. The precise alloy composition of the gold varies according to the dental service conditions [World Gold Council].

Composite resins composed of an organic polymer, which is reinforced by hard particles of silica, were first introduced 40 years ago [Bowen, 1963]. Since then the popularity and variety of composite dental resins has continued to increase. Typical composite resin used includes a monomer of dimethacrylate with fillers such as silane coated ceramic particles. The composite resin is processed as a paste, which is then cured (hardened) with the aid of light after filling. One of the major disadvantages associated with the composite resins is their poor wear resistance. Another disadvantage with the resins is their tendency to shrink during curing leaving gaps. This requires use of other materials and methods to close the gaps that are created during curing.

Aesthetic tooth filling/restorations could be achieved with the use of silicate cements. These cements form when phosphoric acid displaces metal ions from the glass made from alumina silica and other metal oxides. These are known as glass ionomers and have been in use for the past two decades. The setting of these cements is facilitated by the use of polymeric acids which also undergo ionic reactions with Apatite (Calcium phosphate).

Glass ionomer cements offer the possibility of fluoride release into the mouth, bond strongly to teeth and have a similar coefficient of thermal expansion to the tooth enamel [Yap et al., 2000]. Glass ionomers are excessively brittle and research is underway to develop blends of glass ionomers with other materials to improve toughness [Yap, Teo and Teoh, 2000]. A significant convenience in the use of organic composite resins is the use of a strong light source to cause in-situ hardening of the resin. This process is known as photo-polymerization and allows the surgeon to manipulate the resin in an unhurried manner until the resin is ready to be set hard. Setting of the resin is associated with reduction in size (curing shrinkage). This shrinkage can cause the patient post-operative pain and lead to fissures formation between the shrunken resin and tooth cavity. Caries (dental decay) then recurs as bacteria can colonise the shrinkage fissures [Yap, Siow and Ng, Sakaguchi et al., 1992]. One of the typical disadvantages of glass ionomers like the earlier mentioned polymer resins are their poor strength and wear resistance. Current trends in materials development involve the use of organic resins in combination with glass ionomers to overcome this limitation. An important characteristic of any newly developed resin, e.g. a methacrylate polymer, is minimal curing shrinkage [Chung et al., 2002]. The formation of shrinkage cracks after photo-curing is illustrated schematically in Figure 6.2.

The resin material should be inert but in practice may exert side-effects on human tissues. Methyl methacrylate resins are associated with vasodilation (enlargement of blood vessels, such as capillaries) and may lead to pathological conditions in dental patients [Maddux et al., 2002].

6.6   Restorations, orthodontic and periodontic materials

Titanium metallic frameworks form implant-supported restorations, which are cast to improve the fit between the framework and the abutments. A typical problem associated with this practice is rigid anchoring to the bone in the case of osseo-integrated implants, thus restricting later modifications.   Titanium is also used for partial removable dentures as they are lighter compared to Cobalt – Chromium or Gold alloys.   The advantage of using partially removable dentures made of titanium is their bio-compatibility and non-allergenic nature, thus resulting in minimal discomfort to the patients.   Titanium meshes and mini plates are also used in maxillofacial surgery for providing rigid support to bone fragments to help healing.

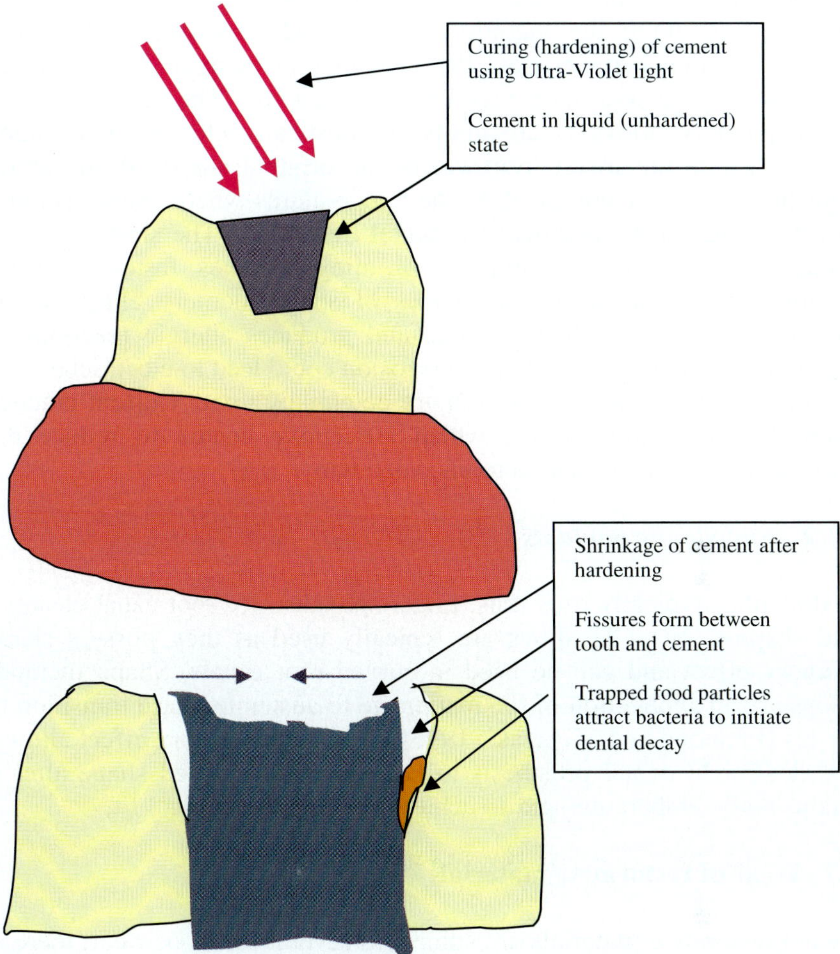

Fig 6.2. Crack formation in filler cements after curing.

6.6.1 *Orthodontic implants*

Orthodontic implants include brackets and arch wire, which are used for tooth alignment and for improving the aesthetics. The most widely used materials include stainless steel and Titanium–Nickel shape memory alloy. Super elastic Nickel- Titanium alloys or Titanium are used for aligning unfavourably positioned teeth or the jaw itself. Initial medical practice used stainless steel wires, which were flexible, the major disadvantage being the inability to withstand very large deflections. Nickel-Titanium wires possess the advantage of being a shape memory alloy, which can withstand very large deflections. The vital feature of shape memory alloys is an ability to drastically change shape upon heating where the metal 'remembers' its original shape. With careful adjustment of alloy composition the temperatures where shape memory effects occur can be practical for dental treatments. The shape memory effect displayed by Titanium-Nickel alloys enables faster teeth re-alignment. One of the disadvantages of shape memory alloys is the presence of Nickel, which is toxic and produces allergic reactions as discussed in Chapter 3. Galvanic corrosion could lead to electrochemical reactions releasing Ni ions, which are potentially toxic. Current practice uses Nickel-Titanium wires, which are epoxy coated to reduce the corrosion potential compared to uncoated wires.

6.6.2 *Endodontic implants*

Endodontics typically uses files, finger spreaders for root canal cleaning and shaping. Ni – Ti alloys are typically used as they possess shape memory effect and can be used in curved root canals. Shape memory alloys are an application of the martensite to austenite phase transition in metals [Fremond and Miyazaki, 1996]. The shape-memory effect allows, e.g., a straight dental prosthesis to later assume a curved shape after it attains body temperature and so achieve a better mechanical fit.

6.7 Wear of restorative materials

Dental restorative materials are subject to several forms of wear, there is direct wear between implants on opposing teeth and third-body wear involving trapped food during mastication. Mechanical fatigue of the filler material by tooth loading is observed to accelerate wear [Yap, Teoh and Chew, 2000].   Thermal fatigue of the implant material may also have a significant accelerating effect on wear, depending on the filler material [Yap, Wee, Teoh and Chew, 2000]. Thermal fatigue occurs whenever a hot drink is imbibed; the filler can be heated to approximately 60 degrees Celsius before cooling to body temperature. Wearing contact between teeth, which is called occlusal contact is often the most aggressive cause of filler wear [Yap, Teoh and Chew, 2000].

This is largely due to the high contact stresses involved in occlusal contact where a contact stress of 20 MPa is typical. The mechanism of occlusal contact is illustrated schematically in Figure 6.3

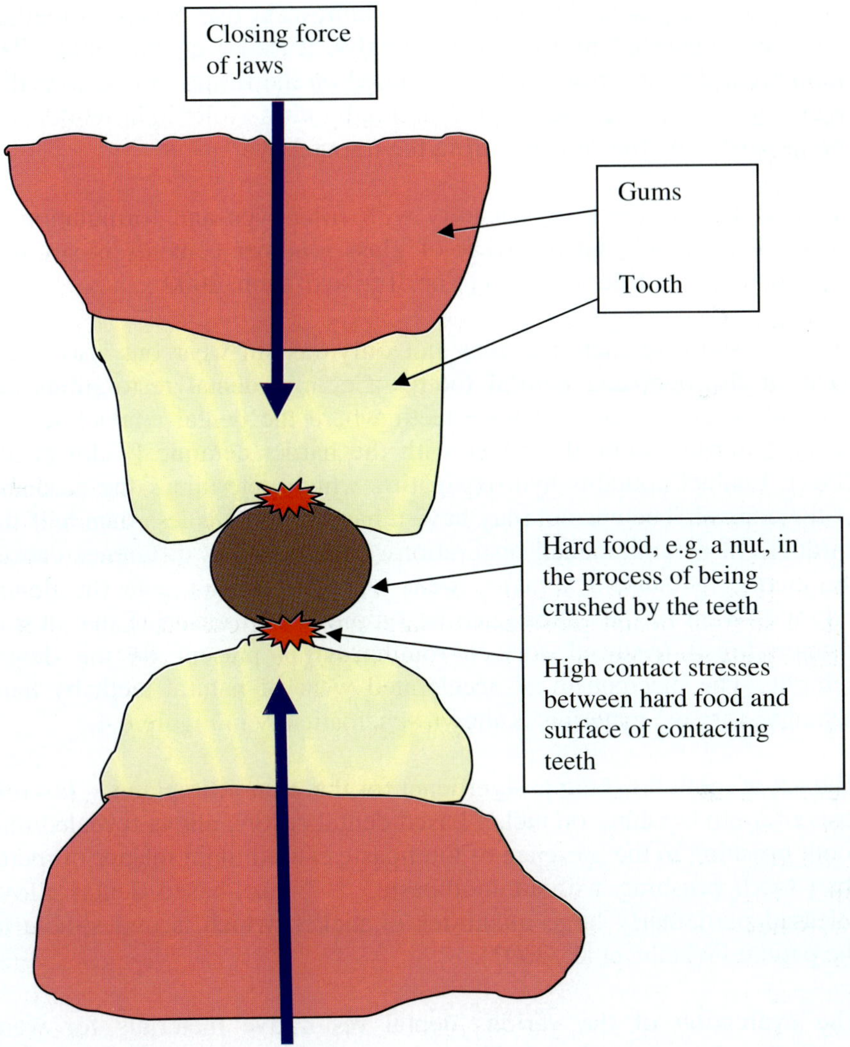

Fig 6.3. Mechanism of high stresses generated by occlusal contact between opposing teeth.

Wear is associated with micro-fracture at the surface of the dental implant, especially at the margin between the restorative material and the surrounding tooth. Ceramic restorations are especially vulnerable, in service fracture being caused by micro-cracks that were inadvertently generated during manufacture. The detection of these microcracks presents much practical difficulty, the fluorescent dye penetrant method has been suggested as the most effective [Fischer et al., 2002]. The fluorescent dye penetrant method is based on the filling of cracks with a liquid dye by capillary action. Irradiation by ultra-violet light renders the cracks visible by fluorescence from the trapped dye.

Wear of fillers varies significantly with filler type and formulation of fillers. It is found that the wear of glass ionomer cements is strongly dependent on the filler material [Yap, Teo and Teoh, 2000].

Dental restorative materials may not only sustain wear but also cause wear of the opposing natural tooth. Ceramic dental restorations are associated with wear of natural teeth where the dental enamel suffers damage during occlusal contact with the harder ceramic [Kalin et al., 2002]. Enamel contains hydroxyapatite, which determines the hardness of the enamel. The enamel may have a hardness that is less than half the hardness of ceramic dental restorations. This hardness difference causes the enamel to sustain abrasive wear when in contact with the dental ceramic. Wear of the enamel can be suppressed by ensuring that, a fine surface finish (reduced surface roughness) is present on the dental ceramic. The mechanism of accelerated wear of natural teeth by hard dental restorative materials is shown schematically in Figure 6.4.

The act of tooth brushing is significant for the wear of implants. In-vitro tests of tooth brushing on nickel-based dental casting alloys revealed that tooth brushing in the presence of toothpaste caused more release of metal than tooth brushing without toothpaste. Nickel-based dental alloys released particularly large quantities of nickel, which is undesirable to the patient [Wataha et al., 2003].

The evaluation of the various dental restorative materials for wear resistance is a complex task. An accepted method is the clinical monitoring of patients but this involves the difficulties such as the irregularity of patients' visits to the clinic, variability in eating and mastication habits and variations in the pH of the saliva [Bianchi et al., 2000]. A new test procedure and apparatus to assess the abrasive wear resistance of dental restorative materials under conditions resembling that of the human mouth has recently been devised [Bianchi et al., 2002] and shown to produce a consistent evaluation of the implant material. It should be noted that unless a wear test closely simulates conditions in the human mouth, the measured wear resistance might not correlate with the wear resistance in service.

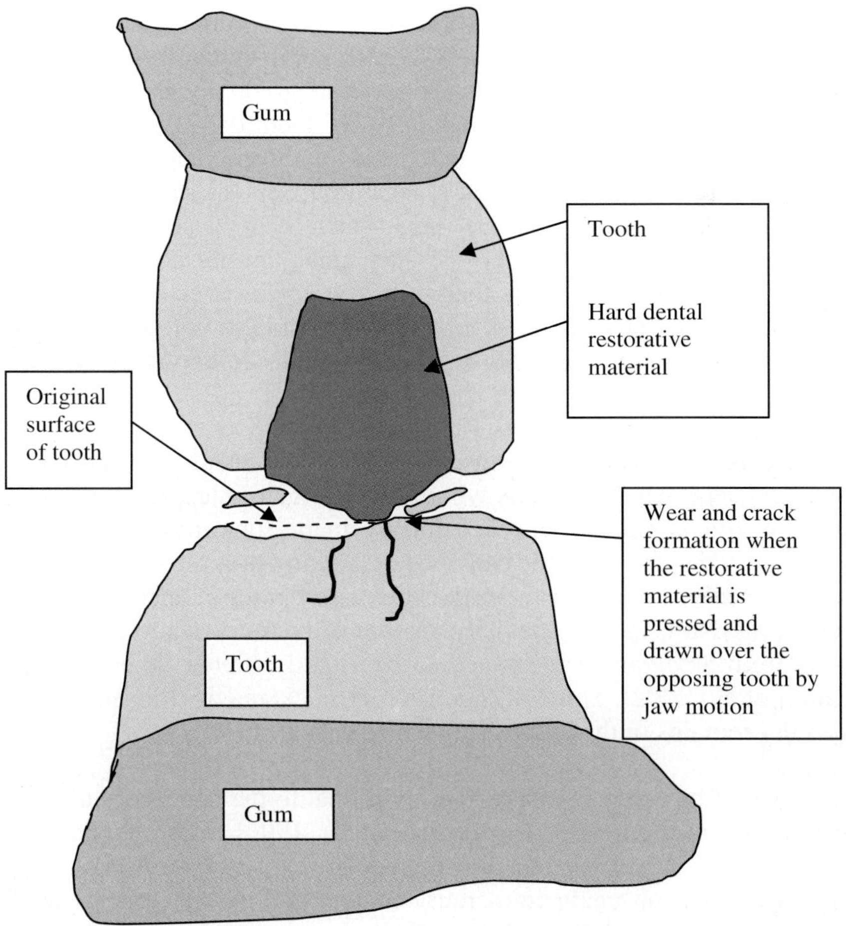

Fig 6.4. Mechanism of wear in a natural tooth by a harder opposing dental restorative material.

6.8   Corrosion behavior of dental restorative materials

Dental implants are exposed to a combination of saliva and atmospheric oxygen, and some electrochemical corrosion of metal implants is almost certain to occur. The grinding of food and opposing teeth against the implant surface would cause corrosive-wear of the metal implant.

6.8.1   *Metal amalgam restorative materials*

A common type of restorative material is the mercury amalgam filling, which is used for dental fillings. The amalgam is composed of primarily mercury, silver, copper and tin. The mercury amalgam was originally proposed in 1826 in France, as a paste that gradually hardened [Null, 1992]. In the late 19th Century and early 20th Century, mercury amalgam gained acceptance from dental societies as a cheaper substitute for gold fillings [Null, 1992]. In recent years, concerns about the effect of mercury leakage on the patients' health have been raised [Guzzi et al., 2002]. The other metals in the mercury amalgam are considered to be less significant as risk factors than mercury.   However, higher strength restorative materials such as crowns and bridges will contain other metals such as aluminium and beryllium, which are known to be highly toxic [Null, 1992].

The complex mixture of metals in an amalgam would be expected to generate electrochemical cells within the amalgam microstructure. These electrochemical cells would then release metal ions into the contacting saliva or juices from masticated food. The corrosion of dental amalgam is estimated to release in the order of 1 microgram of mercury per day per filling [Null, 1992]. The daily amount of mercury adsorption into the body from amalgam is estimated to be slightly higher than this figure [Guzzi et al., 2002]. Some of this mercury is excreted while some of the mercury remains in the tissues [Lorscheider et al. 1995].

The level of mercury exposure is proportional to the number of amalgam restorations in the mouth [Lorscheider et al., 1995], where a patient has many amalgam restorations, a high mercury exposure may result. Significant loss of amalgam mercury content is found in some 5 and 10-year old fillings [Null, 1992].   Bacteria in the mouth can convert mercury into methyl-mercury, which is yet more toxic than elemental mercury [Guzzi et al., 2002].

Elemental mercury is not only lost from the amalgam by corrosion, it also escapes by volatilization. It is estimated that the concentration of mercury vapour in the mouth may become sufficiently high to be toxic [Null, 1992]. Mercury vapour can then enter the body via the lungs during inspiration (breathing in). The volatilization of mercury is significantly increased by the mastication (chewing) of food, which presumably activates the surface of the amalgam by mechanical abrasion [Otto et al. 1986; Bjorkman and Lind, 1992]. An ameliorating factor is the film of saliva, which usually covers the teeth and the fillings. The thickness of the saliva film on the teeth and inner surfaces of the mouth ranges from 70 to 100 micrometres [Collins and Dawes, 1987] and this is found to act as a major barrier to the escape of mercury. Model tests with artificial saliva films of about 140 micrometres thickness on previously abraded amalgam specimens revealed a 10 to 100-fold reduction mercury emissions compared to dry abraded amalgam [Mahler et al., 2002]. This reduction in mercury emissions is far greater than would occur if the saliva film acted as a simple diffusion barrier. Information on the mercury concentration on the artificial saliva is not available, so it is not clear whether the mercury was retained in the amalgam or whether it was merely diverted into the simulated liquid saliva. Studies of mercury levels in natural saliva have shown that the presence of amalgam restorative materials raises the level of mercury in the saliva beyond that found in patients without amalgam restorations [Leistevuo et al., 2001]. This finding implies that mercury is released from the amalgam into the saliva. The mechanisms of degradation of restorative materials such as mercury amalgam fillings are illustrated schematically in Figure 6.5.

The issue of mercury loss from amalgam restorative materials and its effect on human health remains controversial. The American Dental Association has stated that dental amalgam is a safe and valuable material for dental treatment [American Dental Association, 2002]. A fundamental issue is whether substitutes for amalgam are actually safer. Substitute metals and organic compounds have been found to present health risks also [Folwaczny and Hickel, 2002]. At the time of writing, clinical trials by the US National Institutes of Health on the effect of dental amalgam remains incomplete [Larkin, 2002].

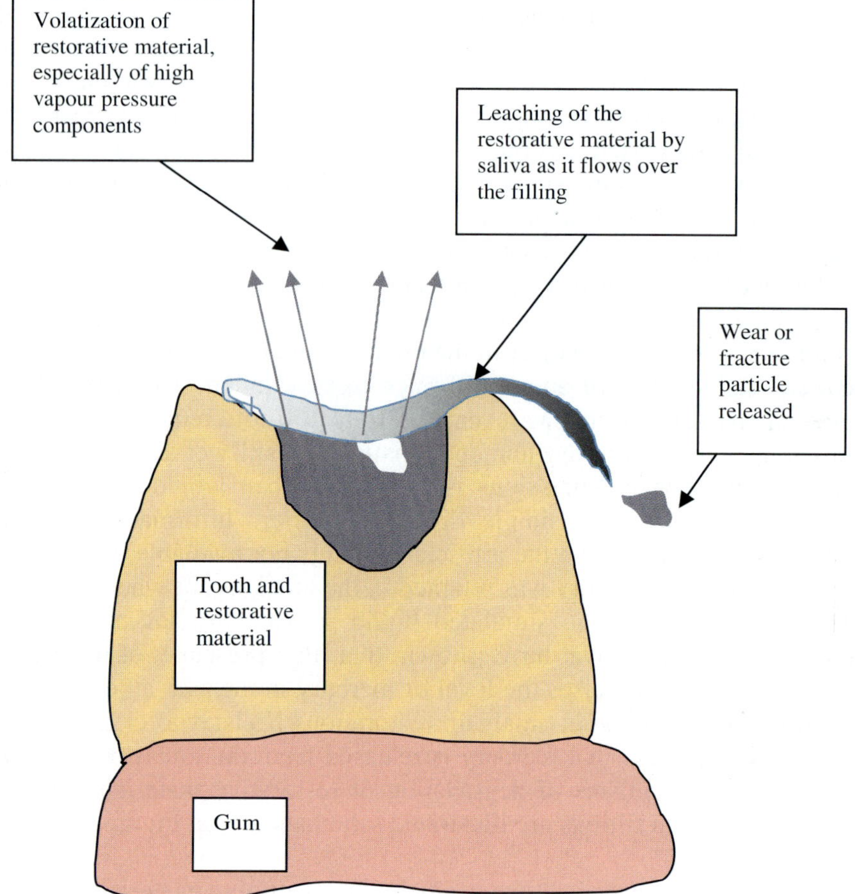

Fig 6.5. Mechanisms of degradation of dental restorative materials.

6.8.2 *Ceramic and polymer restorative materials*

Ceramic materials are much more resistant to electrochemical corrosion than metals and the white luster of ceramics closely resembles natural teeth than the shine from a metal surface. Ceramics are prone to a corrosive phenomenon known as ion leakage, where ions of e.g., aluminium, are released from the ionic crystal lattice. *In vitro* tests of glassy and crystalline ceramic specimens in 4% acetic acid at 80 degrees

Celsius revealed substantial ion leaching of most of the constituent metal ions in the glass, such as sodium, potassium, magnesium and yttrium. Silicon was also lost from the ceramic in these tests [Milleding et al. 2002]. Glassy ceramics were found to lose ions more rapidly than crystalline ceramics. The relationship between these in vitro tests and ion leaching inside the human mouth remains largely unexplored.

Polymer implant materials, such as acrylic resins are not immune to water damage. Water solubility, or the lack of it, is an important service characteristic of methacrylate polymer cements [Chung et al., 2002]. The wet conditions inside the human mouth also affect the setting (polymerization) of polymer cements. Segregation between the hydrophilic (water-attracting) and hydrophobic (water-repelling) components of the polymer resin may occur [Spencer and Wang, 2002]. This segregation leads to the formation of an undesirable porous structure close to the interface between dentin and resin [Spencer and Wang, 2002].

6.9 Summary

Various dental restorative materials and endodontic tools are reviewed in brief. Emphasis is given to oral implants and restorative materials, which are most commonly encountered in dentistry. Various materials are used in oral implants such as dental amalgams for fillers, endosteal, sub-periosteal implants. Most dental restorative materials suffer from at least one form of materials degradation such as wear or corrosion leading to concerns about the release of toxic substances. Titanium alloys are widely used in all the divisions of dentistry such as oral, maxillofacial, prosthodontics and orthodontics owing to their biocompatibility and non allergenic nature. Polymer materials are becoming useful as restorative materials as improvements in toughness and wear resistance accrue.

References

American Dental Association, ADA Statement on dental amalgam, 8th January, 2002,
http://www.ada.org/prof/resources/ positions/statements/amalgam.asp

E.C. Bianchi, E.J. da Silva, R.D. Monici, C.A. de Freitas and A.R.R. Bianchi, Development of new standard procedures for the evaluation of dental composite abrasive wear, Wear, 2002, Vol. 253, pp. 533-540.

L. Bjorkman and B. Lind, Factors influencing mercury evaporation rate from dental amalgam fillings, Scandinavian Journal of Dental Research, 1992, Vol. 100, pp. 354-360.

R.L. Bowen, Properties of silica reinforced polymer for dental restorations, Journal of American Dental Association, 1963, Vol. 66, No. 1, pp. 57-64.

C.-M. Chung, M.-S. Kim, J.-G. Kim and D.-O. Jang, Synthesis and photopolymerization of trifunctional methacrylates and their application as dental monomers, Journal of Biomedical Materials Research, 2002, Vol. 62, No. 4, pp. 622-627.

L.M. Collins and C. Dawes, The surface area of the adult human mouth and the thickness of the salivary film covering the teeth and oral mucosa, Journal of Dental Research, 1987, Vol. 66, pp. 1300-1302.

X.D. Dong and N.D. Ruse, Fatigue crack propagation path across the dentinoenamel junction complex in human teeth, Journal of Biomedical Materials Research Part A, 2003, Vol. 66A, No. 1, pp. 103-109.

Matthias Folwaczny and Reinhard Hickel, *Correspondence to 'Should amalgam fillings be removed?'*, The Lancet, 21 December 2002, Vol. 360, No. 9350.

M. Fremond and S. Miyazaki, Shape Memory Alloys, 1996, publ. Springer-Verlag, Heidelberg, Germany.

J. Gabrovsek (4) , Dental caries: a dent on dogma, part 4, <u>Dentistry On-Line</u>, Priory Lodge Education Ltd, 1997, <u>http://www.pol-it.org/den/caries04.htm</u>

J.Gabrovsek (3), Dental caries: a dent on dogma, part 3, <u>Dentistry On-Line</u>, Priory Lodge Education Ltd, 1997, <u>http://www.pol-it.org/den/caries03.htm</u>

J. Gabrovsek (2), Dental caries: a dent on dogma, part 2, <u>Dentistry On-Line</u>, Priory Lodge Education Ltd, 1997, <u>http://www.pol-it.org/den/caries02.htm</u>

Glossary of Prosthodontic Terms, 6th edition, Journal of Prosthetic Dentistry, Vol. 71, No. 1, pp. 41-112.

B. Groessner-Schreiber, A. Neubert, W.-D. Muller, M. Hopp, M. Griepentrog and K.-P. Lange, Fibroblast growth on surface-modified dental implants: An in vitro study, Journal of Biomedical Materials Research, 2003, Vol. 64A, No. 4, pp. 591-599.

Gianpaolo Guzzi, Marco Grandi and Cristina Cattaneo, *Correspondence to 'Should amalgam fillings be removed?'*, The Lancet, 21 December 2002, Vol. 360, No. 9350.

Junther Heinke and Cornelius . G . Wittal.Osseointegrated dental implants – follow up studies, Biomaterials engineering and devices, Human applications Vol II. Orthopeadic, dental and bone graft applications, Humana press,2000, pp. - 67- 92.

Mitjan Kalin, Said Jahanmir and Lewis K. Ives, Effect of counterface roughness on abrasive wear of hydroxyapatite, **Wear**, 2002, Vol. 252, pp. 679-685.

Burton Langer and William Becker, Osseointegration and treatment planning - Periodontists perspectives, The Branemark Osseointegrated implant, Edited Tomas Albrektsson and George A. Zarb, Quintessence Publishing Co. Inc., 1989 pp. –127-138.

Marilynn Larkin, Don't remove amalgam fillings, urges American Dental Association, *'Science and Medicine'*, The Lancet, 3 August 2002, Vol. 360, No. 9330.

J. Leistevuo, T. Leistevuo, H. Helnius, L. Pyy, R. Huovinena and J. Tenuvuob, Dental amalgam fillings and the amount of organic mercury in human saliva, Caries research, 2001, Vol. 35, No. 3, pp. 163-166.

J.P. Ley, A.N. Cranin, M. Katzap, Biomaterials used in in Implant Dentistry, Biomaterials Engineering and Devices: Human Applications, Vol.2., Orthopaedic, Dental and Bone Graft Applications, edit. Donald. L. Wise, Debra J. Trantolo, Kai-Uwe Lewandrowski, Joseph D. Gresser, Mario V. Cattaneo and Michael J. Yaszemski, Human Press, 2000, Totowa, New Jersey, USA, pp. 3-24.

H. Li and Z.R. Zhou, Wear behaviour of human teeth in dry and artificial saliva conditions, Wear, 2002, Vol. 249, pp. 980-984.

F.L. Lorscheider, M.J. Vimy and B. Lind, Mercury concentrations in the human brain and kidneys in relation to exposure from dental amalgam fillings, FASEB Journal, 1995, Vol. 9, pp. 504-508.

Z.-X. Luo, R.L. Cifelli and Z. Kielan-Jaworowska, Dual origin of tribosphenic mammals, Nature, 2001, Vol. 409, pp. 53-57.

Gemalloy, Technical data.,
http://www.syriagate.com/gemalloy /amalgam.htm

D.B. Mahler, J.D. Adey, L.E. Simms and M. Marek, Influence of liquid films on mercury vapor loss from dental amalgam, Dental Materials, 2002, Vol. 18, pp. 407-412.

J. Mau, A. Behneke, N. Behneke, C.U. Fritzemeier, G. Gomez-Roman, B. d'Hoedt, H. Spiekermann, V. Strunz and M. Yong, Randomized multicenter comparison of two coatings of intramobile cylinder implants in 313 partially edentulous mandibles followed up for 5 years, Clinical Oral Implants Research, 2002, Vol. 13, No. 5, pp. 477-487.

L.M. Macpherson, T.W. MacFarlane, K.W. Stephen, An intra-oral study of the plaque microflora associated with early enamel demineralization. Journal of Dental Research, 1990, Vol. 69, No. 11, pp 1712-6.

Macro Esposito, Ti in dental applications (I), Ti in medicine, material science, surface science, Engineering, Biological responses and Medical applications, Ed. D.M. Brunette et al, Springer Verlag Publ. 2001, pp. 827 – 873.
www.Titaniuminmedicine.com

P. Milleding, C. Haraldsson and S. Karlsson, Ion leaching from dental ceramics during static in vitro corrosion testing, Journal of Biomedical Materials Research, 2002, Vol. 61, No. 4, pp. 541-550.

G. Null, Mercury Dental Amalgams, Analyzing the debate, Townsend Letter or Doctors August/ September 1992, http://www.garynull.com/documents/MercuryDentalAmalgams.htm

J.L. Ong, C.N.D. Chan, K. Bessho, HA Coatings on Dental Implants, Biomaterials Engineering and Devices: Human Applications, Vol.2., Orthopaedic, Dental and Bone Graft Applications, edit. Donald. L. Wise, Debra J. Trantolo, Kai-Uwe Lewandrowski, Joseph D. Gresser, Mario V. Cattaneo and Michael J. Yaszemski, Human Press, 2000, Totowa, New Jersey, USA, pp. 49-60.

K.H. Ott, T. Krafft, A. Kroncke, K.H. Schaller, H. Valentin and D. Weltle, Duration of mercury release from amalgam fillings after chewing, Deutsche Zahnartzliche Zeitschrift, 1986, Vol. 41, pp. 968-72.

R.L. Sakaguchi, W.H. Douglas and R.B. Peters, Curing light performance and polymerization of composite restorative materials, Journal of Dentistry, 1992, Vol. 20, pp. 183-188.

D. Skrtic, J.M. Antonucci and E.D. Eanes, Amorphous calcium phosphate-based bioactive polymeric composites for mineralized tissue regeneration, Journal of Research of the National Institute of Standards and Technology, 2003, Vol. 108, pp. 167-183.

J. Shackleton, Evolution: Poles apart, molars together, Nature Science update, Thursday 4 January 2001.

P. Spencer and Y. Wang, Adhesive phase separation at the dentin interface under wet bonding conditions, Journal of Biomedical Materials Research, 2002, Vol. 62, No. 3, pp. 447-456.

P. Spyrou, S. Papaioannou, G. Hampson, K. Brady, R.M. Palmer and F. McDonald, Cytokine release by osteoblast-like cells cultured on implanted discs of varying alloy compositions, Clinical Oral Implants Research, 2002, Vol. 13, No. 6, pp. 623-630.

The Hindu, 2003, http://www.hinduonnet.com/thehindu/mag/2003/03/16/stories/2003031600200700.htm

Diane B. Wayne, Cynthia P. Trajtenberg, David J. Hyman Tooth and Periodontal Disease: A Review for the Primary-Care Physician, Southern Medical Journal 94(9):925-932, 2001.

Peter Thompson, Ti and inflammatory response, The Branemark Osseointegrated implant, Edited by Tomas Albrektsson and George A. Zarb, Quintessence Publishing Co. Inc., 1989 pp. – 25 -35.

Gean Francois Tulasne, Implant treatment of missing posterior dentition, The Branemark Osseointegrated implant, Edited Tomas Albrektsson and George A. Zarb, Quintessence Publishing Co. Inc., 1989 pp. –103-115.

J.C. Wataha, P.E. Lockwood, D. Mettenburg and S. Bouillaguet, Toothbrushing causes elemental release from dental casting alloys, Journal of Biomedical Materials Research Part B, Applied Biomaterials, 2003, Vol. 65B, No. 1, pp. 180-185.

World Gold Council, Industrial and Dental Uses of Gold. http://www.gold.org/Ginfos/Gi8ind.htm

A.U.J Yap, J.C.M. Teo and S.H. Teoh, Comparative wear resistance of restorative reinforced glass ionomer cements, Proc. 10th International Conference on Biomedical Engineering, 6-9 December 2000, Singapore, edit. JCH Goh, publ. National University of Singapore, page 604.

A.U.J. Yap, K.S. Siow and S.C. Ng, Soft-start polymerization: influence of effectiveness of cure and post-gel shrinkage, Proc. 10th International Conference on Biomedical Engineering, 6-9 December 2000, Singapore, edit. JCH Goh, publ. National University of Singapore, page 587.

A.U.J. Yap, S.H. Teoh and C.L. Chew, Effects of cyclic loading on occlusal contact area wear of composite restoratives, Proc. 10th International Conference on Biomedical Engineering, 6-9 December

2000, Singapore, edit. JCH Goh, publ. National University of Singapore, pp. 323-324.

A.U.J. Yap, K.E.C. Wee, S.H. Teoh and C.L. Chew, Influence of thermal fatigue on OCA wear of composite restoratives, Proc. 10th International Conference on Biomedical Engineering, 6-9 December 2000, Singapore, edit. JCH Goh, publ. National University of Singapore, pp. 325-326.

George A. Zarb, Impact of osseointegration on pre-prosthetic surgery, The Branemark Osseointegrated implant, Edited Tomas Albrektsson and George A. Zarb, Quintessence Publishing Co. Inc., 1989, pp. 91-102.

Chapter 7

Bioartificial Pancreas and Bioartificial Liver

7.1 Introduction

Artificial organs are similar to conventional implants since they are placed within the human body to closely fit into and support natural tissues. However, artificial organs are different from implants, which are only intended to perform a passive structural role, whereas the artificial organ is expected to perform an active biochemical function

Research into artificial organs has developed rapidly in recent years, with predictions of clinically usable artificial organs being ready within a decade. The term 'artificial organs' is accessible but imprecise because it is not the intention to try and reproduce natural organs in all their complexity. Instead, systems that are much simpler in shape and function are being developed with the purpose of remedying some pathological condition.

Since artificial organs are still in their infancy, there is hardly any information on their long-term service characteristics. Long-term service characteristics will become an important question, since artificial organs will inevitably be expected to reliably perform for periods similar to those expected of orthopaedic endoprostheses (artificial joints). In this chapter, artificial organs to treat diabetes and liver disease are discussed. These are diseases, which are often present as a chronic long-term problem in advanced societies.

7.2 Diabetes and liver disease

Diabetes mellitus and chronic liver diseases are among the main causes for medical complications in patients and mortality. Medical Research has been directed to find a solution to these problems. The advances in tissue engineering and cell biology have assisted the development of bio artificial organs as the potential alternative treatment method. Over the past two decades tissue engineering has seen significant developments and uses cell biology and material science and engineering for developing biological substitutes for repair and regeneration of a tissue or an organ function. Bio artificial liver and pancreas have important functions in the human system for digestion and maintaining a balance of the sugars in the human body. Liver failure can be classified into two categories, namely fulminant liver failure and chronic liver disease, which require transplant of liver. Similarly pancreatic failure can lead to decrease in insulin secretion resulting in abnormal blood sugar levels in patients. This is termed as diabetes and can be classified into two categories namely type I and type II diabetes. Type I diabetes is caused by environmental and genetic factors that results in complete absence or lack of essential amount of insulin required for converting the sugar into useful components while type II diabetes is mainly caused by obesity necessitating medications and at times injection of insulin. Insulin secretion can be brought to necessary limits with suitable diet and exercise in case of patients with type II diabetes. An alternative treatment method for patients with Type I diabetes is the use of artificial pancreas.

7.3 Pancreas and liver

Pancreas and liver forms important organs in humans for performing definite functions such as control of blood sugar and secretion of juices to assist digestion respectively. Malfunctioning of these devices can lead to many complications in patients and finally morbidity. Pancreas is a lobulated gland situated in the upper abdomen and secretes digestive juices. The hormones released are delivered to the liver. Pancreatic islets consist of alpha cells and beta cells. The alpha cell is located at the periphery while the beta cells occupy the center of the islets. The alpha cells act as a source of glucagon, a hormone inducing the liver to release glucose, and the acids. Beta cells secrete insulin to sequestrate carbohydrate, protein and fat in the storage depots of liver muscle and the tissues. Artificial pancreas refers to replacing endocrine functions of pancreatic islets. This does not necessarily mean the complete replacement of exocrine function, which includes the digestive components of pancreas besides the endocrine function (insulin secretion). Insulin deficiency as explained earlier is a life threatening condition and so much of the development of the bio-artificial pancreas is directed to insulin supply systems. The insulin deficiency known as diabetes mellitus has affected many people around the world. The treatment methods include constant administration of drugs and injection of insulin at frequent intervals (daily or weekly basis). The composition of insulin varies between the species e.g. human and animal. Insulin cannot be taken orally, as it would be digested in the gastro-intestinal tract thus necessitating intravenous administration (injections). Since insulin is active for short duration, regular injections are necessary in patients with type I diabetes and this causes discomfort in patients. This lead to the development of implantable reservoirs made of silicone elastomer with a delivery catheter that can be refilled. The insulin in the reservoir is made to drain at a constant rate into the peritoneal cavity. This concept has a serious disadvantage of producing tissue reactions and infection. Furthermore biological deposits may also obstruct the delivery catheter.   There is also a risk of over-dose of insulin due to accidental rupture or other malfunction.

Considering the deficiencies of the insulin delivery systems discussed, insulin pumps, housing of which is made of titanium, were developed which could be implanted into the patients. These pumps could be preprogrammed to have adjustable flow rates. However, pumps do have certain restrictions with respect to acceptance by the surrounding tissue and replenishment of the insulin after the therapy or after exhaustion of the attached insulin reservoir.

In view of the problems associated with external insulin supply devices, research was directed towards insulin production systems in which the insulin can be synthesized and released/secreted as needed on demand. Pancreatic transplantation was attempted as a part of this motive and human allograph transplantation was tried to deal with endocrine gland secretion. One of the key restricting factors to this attempt was identification of healthy organs and donors acceptance in patients. Human islet transplantation, have gained importance owing to clinical demonstration of insulin independence in type I diabetic patients. Autologous islet transplantation have been performed in patients with polycystic disease (tumors, trauma etc).

Bio artificial pancreas produced insulin to regulate glycemia combining the beta cells with the synthetic polymer membrane. For glucose tolerance, large number of islets is required and sourcing of these for human islet transplantation may be difficult. To overcome these limitations, porcine islets are favored compared to bovine islets, due to similarity between the human and porcine insulin.

One of the problems associated with islet transplant is immuno-rejective reaction by the surrounding tissue leading to antibody production and destruction of the islets. To overcome this limitation immuno suppressive drugs are to be administrated for the rest of the life, which can cause further complications affecting other organs. The method to overcome this problem is immuno isolation of allogeneic or xenogeneic islets.

7.4 Immuno-isolation

An effective method to overcome or eliminating the immuno-suppressive drugs is the use of immuno- isolation devices. Encapsulation of islets in such devices eliminates the need for immuno- suppressive drugs. These isolation devices allow the use of both allografts and xenograft besides autografts and syngeneic (genetically identical individuals) grafts. Here, auto and allografts refer to transplantation from the same species e.g. the patient himself or a suitable donor while xenografts refer to transplants from animal cells/tissues. The immuno – isolation device consists of a semi permeable membrane, which permits low molecular weight substances to be exchanged across the membrane thus effectively shielding them against antibodies or immunocytes. Immuno isolation can be achieved by two methods, such as micro encapsulation or macro encapsulation. In micro-encapsulation, each islet, a gel surrounds Cell cluster or tissue fragment. This cell is made of biocompatible polymer such as calcium alginate, which has semi-permeability. To prevent the degradation of the polymer, it is usually surrounded by a poly-anion.

Macro-encapsulation refers to a larger prefabricated envelope where the slurry of islets is delivered prior to the implantation. The envelope is a semi-permeable membrane restricting access to antibodies, thus protecting the islets. The concept of immuno-isolation is illustrated schematically in Figure 7.1.

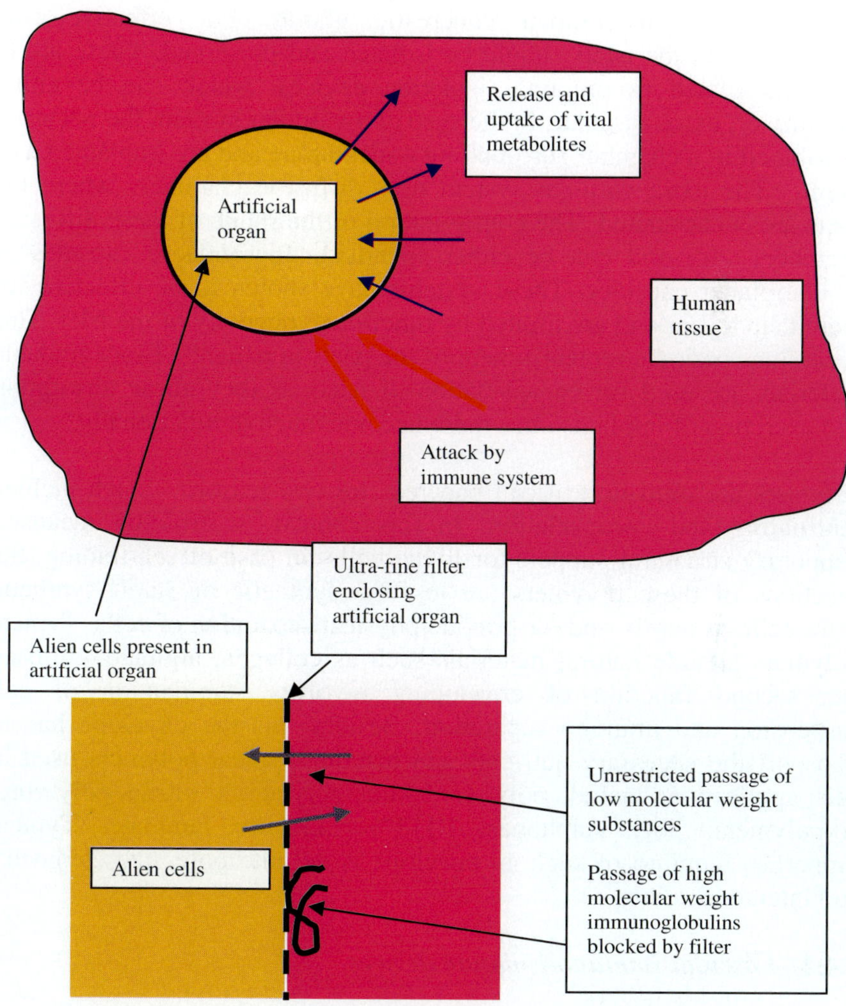

Fig 7.1. Concept of immuno-isolation using a selective filter.

7.4.1 *Islet preservation and encapsulation*

The goal of islet transplantation is to treat patients efficiently in order to have minimum immuno-suppressive drugs. Human pancreatic glands are limited in supply and multiple glands are required for isolating the islets to treat a single patient. This suggests that the technique needs to be improved to use xenografts from animal sources keeping in view the limited supply of human pancreatic glands. For effective islet transplantation the islets should be isolated and preserved. These are to be encapsulated in immuno- isolation devices, which can be either vascular or, extra vascular. In the case of a vascular system, the islets are distributed in a chamber surrounding a membrane and are implanted as a shunt. The extra vascular system uses diffusion chambers where the islets are encapsulated. The configuration or the shape of these diffusion chambers vary and can be either spherical, micro/macro capsules or tubular/planer capsules. These systems have shown to be effective for more than a year and are limited by functional longevity of the islet. This necessities periodic replenishment of the islets in patients. Biodegradable materials are used for encapsulation of islets as they allow absorption and excretion of implants once these become inactive functionally.

Polymers are used in artificial pancreas for two reasons, which include scaffolding and encapsulation. In this context, scaffolding means a temporary structural support for living cells. In case of scaffolding, the functions of these polymers are to form synthetic or semi- synthetic extra-cellular matrix and /or provide physical separation of cells. Typical polymers include natural materials such as collegen, alginate, chitosan etc. second function of enveloping involves stabilization of cell suspension and immuno separation. Besides this the envelope has to transport the necessary nutrients and insulin. Typical polymers used in such applications include poly- L– lysine, poly acrylo nitrile, poly vinyl co-polymers, poly sulphones, PTFE – biopore laminate. Typical properties required of such an envelope is definite pore size, geometry and interconnections.

7.4.2 *Vascular immuno-isolation devices*

As indicated in the earlier paragraph, vascular devices consist of a chamber surrounding the membrane, which possess semi permeability and are used as a shunt in the vascular system. One of the potential problems with such devices is blood clotting. Other critical issues with the use of vascular devices for immuno-isolation include the limitation due to the size and geometry on the islet tissue transplantation. In addition to this, the length of the membrane is limited by the tendency to clot.

7.4.3 *Extravascular immuno-isolation devices*

Due to the limitation with vascular devices, further development resulted in extra vascular chambers being devised for encapsulation of islets. One of the major advantages of these devices is the elimination of the need for major vascular surgery and these chambers were fabricated using biodegradable polymers such as polyacrylonitrile and polyvinylchloride. This permits xenografts such as porcine, bovine, canine islets being transplanted and provided long-term correction of hyperglycemia. Installment of the islet encapsulation device outside of the vascular system permits xenografts such as porcine, bovine and canine islets to be transplanted; long-term correction of hyperglycaemia can also be obtained [Lanza et al.,1991]. Some of the safety issues remaining to be addressed include long-term biocompatibility and the likelihood of membrane failure. Materials used in the membrane of immuno-isolation devices comprise of collagen, gelatin, alginate, agarose, chitosan, hyaluronan and polysulphones, as well as other materials. Further medical problems such as fibrosis, abscess formation and unwanted adhesion to other organs may also be minimized by this implantation method. This design also eliminated the problems such as fibrosis, abscess formation and adhesions. Some of the safety issues yet to be addressed include long-term biocompatibility, membrane failure. Some of the materials used for immuno-isolation devices include collagen, gelatin, alginate, agarose, chitosan, hyaluronan, and polysulphones.

7.5 Bio-reactor for hybrid liver support

Liver is the next important organ to the pancreas, which plays a key role in digestion. In general liver can be classified as a biochemical reactor within the human body, which has multiple functions, which are critical for homeostasis. The liver has the valuable characteristic of regenerating after an episode of tissue damage. Chronic diseases or fulminant liver failure as a result of necrosis of hepatocytes necessitates the use of bio-artificial liver/liver support systems. The mortality rate of fulminant hepatic failure is quite high. On the other hand, chronic hepatic failure is a progressive form of disease due to long standing toxic exposure such as alcoholism or secondary to viral hepatitis. Some of the effects of acute liver failure include cerebral oedema, impaired blood coagulation and hemorrhage in the gastro- intestinal system. Liver transplantation is the most effective procedure for hepatic failures. Orthotopic liver transplantation has been used in case of acute liver failure successfully but the mortality rate continues to be unacceptably high. In order to overcome this lacuna, numerous methods have been investigated whose prime aim is to temporally replace certain functions of the failed liver. The primary intention is to detoxify the toxic products in case of chronic liver failure or to have liver perfusion. The newer system of treatment uses bio artificial or cell based treatment methods. The blood purification method includes haemo dialysis, haemo filtration, haemo dye absorption, plasma pheresis and albumin dialysis.   None of these methods are popular as they do not reduce the morbidity or mortality in patients. *Ex vivo* perfusion is one of the methods used in patients with liver failure, which primarily have extra-corporeal liver perfusion. In this method a xenogeneic or allogeneic liver is used for perfusing the blood of the patients. This methodology showed better survival rates compared to blood purification systems. The second class of treatment methods includes in vitro bio artificial systems, which could provide a broad array of liver functions. This consists of a liver tissue with a bioreactor in an extra corporeal circuit. The liver tissue/hepatocytes are either from primary human hepatocytes or non-human such as porcine [Ronald et al.,2001]. Non-human cells/ tissues include those from rats, pigs and rabbits. Human cells have an advantage of not triggering or having minimal immune responses. These human cells or tissues are short supply and are not readily available. The advances in cell biology have lead to the maintenance of hepatocytes in vitro. There are different methods of the maintenance of hepatocytes, which include

    (I)   Immobilization of cells on artificial membranes e.g. synthetic polymers

    (II)   Use of artificial bodies to promote cell adhesion.

    (III)   Encapsulation of cells within semi-permeable membranes.

Bioreactors perform a large-scale function of the methods highlighted and these function as a hybrid extracorporeal liver support system.

7.6 Summary

Artificial organs, which are biochemically active systems in close proximity to human tissue, are rapidly developing into an important new method of treatment for problems such as diabetes and liver disease. In time, the long-term service characteristics of the artificial organ will become important to ensure reliable support to patients. The role of biomaterials is to provide a protective framework for natural cells to perform vital metabolic functions in an artificial organ. The source of the natural cells is of considerable concern. Due to the limitations of using autografts (tissue sourced from the same patient) or allografts (tissues sourced from other patients), it is necessary to use xenografts (tissues from animals) such as from pigs. The human immune system is very intolerant of anything but cells from the same body and can initiate a rapid process of destruction of the alien cells. The role of the biomaterial is offer what is known as immuno-isolation, where a filter prevents antibodies and other components of the human immune system from attacking the alien cells in the artificial organ. The filter allows lower molecular weight substances such as sugar to be released from the artificial organ while excluding the higher molecular weight proteins typical of the immune system. The long-term durability of this filter remains an open question for future research.

References

Bioartificial organs III Tissue Sourcing, Immunoisolation and Clinical Trials, Ed. David Hunkeler, Allan Cherrington, Ales Prokop and Ray Rajotte, Annals of New York Academy of Sciences, 2001, Vol. 944, pp. 249-398.

Bioartificial organs II Technology, Medicine and Materials, Ed. David Hunkeler, Ales Prokop, Allan D. Cherrington, Ray V. Rajotte, and Michael Sefton, Annals of New York Academy of Sciences, 1999, Vol. 875, Parts 1-7, pp. 175-254.

Bioartificial organs II Technology, Medicine and Materials, Ed. David Hunkeler, Ales Prokop, Allan D. Cherrington, Ray V. Rajotte, and Michael Sefton, Annals of New York Academy of Sciences, 1999, Vol. 875, Parts 1-7, pp. 310-368.

Bioartificial Organs; Science, Medicine and Technology, Ed. Ales Prokop, David Hunkeler, Allan D. Cherrington, Annals of New York Academy of Sciences, 1997, Vol. 831, pp. 62-186, 226-361.

RP Lanza,   DH Butler,   KM Borland,   JE Staruk,   DL Faustman, BA Solomon,   TE Muller,   RG Rupp,   T Maki,   AP Monaco,   and WL Chick, "Xenotransplantation of Canine, Bovine, and Porcine Islets in Diabetic Rats Without Immunosuppression" , Proc Natl Acad Sci U S A. 1991 December 15; 88 (24): 11100–11104.

Ronald A. Faris, Tamako Konkin, and Gretchen Halpert, Liver Stem Cells: A Potential Source of Hepatocytes for the Treatment of Human Liver Disease, Artificial Organs, 25 Issue 7 Page 513 - July 2001.

The Biomedical Engineering Handbook 2nd edition, Vol. II, Ed. Joseph D Bronzino, 1999,publ. CRC Press, Florida, USA.

Chapter 8

Implants and Biomaterials for External Bodily Functions and Cosmetic Advantage

8.1 Introduction

The human body displays perhaps as much sensitivity to materials, which only contact the exterior of the body, as to those materials implanted within the body This sensitivity is exemplified by the case of an anesthetist, who was virtually forced to change her profession because of acquired sensitization to natural latex gloves in the course of her work. This anaesthetist's strong allergic reaction to natural latex gloves rendered her unable to adequately serve the patient.   Fortunately, the person concerned was able to find satisfaction and reward in another profession [Larkin, 2001]. Biocompatibility is therefore of critical importance to designers of devices and systems for external bodily functions.

Another more widespread but less acute example of pathological reaction to handled materials is the case of the new Euro coin, which causes dermatitis in susceptible individuals. The problem is the Euro coin is composed of two alloys, which form a galvanic couple when handled by a sweaty hand. Sweat is largely composed of saline solution, which is an efficient electrolyte. Galvanic corrosion then ensures which releases nickel ions. Approximately 30% of the populations are sensitive to nickel ions, suffering various allergic effects [Nestle et al., 2002].

Latex products may also create risks even for the majority of the population who are not allergic to this material.   Residual bacteria lodged on the surface of latex products such as gloves and catheters may generate a fever in users even when the latex product has been thoroughly sterilized by gamma-radiation [Haishima et al. 2001]. The reason for this is that the killed bacteria still contain endotoxins, which become pyrogenic (cause fevers) after contamination of the user.   A mechanism of contamination, used in the cited research, is water-borne transfer from the surface of the latex to the tissues of the animal or human subject.

Another important characteristic of rubber gloves is resistance to mechanical fatigue when the gloved fingers are flexed.   Failure under mechanical fatigue allows microorganisms such as viruses to penetrate the glove. It was found that chlorinated gloves showed a reduced fatigue life compared to unchlorinated gloves, both powdered and unpowdered gloves [Scwherin et al., 2002].

8.2   Opthalmic implants and contact lenses

Several conditions such as macular hole, diabetic retinopathy, mypoia, astigmatism, hyperopia, macular edema etc can require either corrective surgical technique or use of biomaterials to repair or restore functionality of the eye. Retinal tear or retinal detachment is one of the important conditions that require treatment or corrective surgical procedure to restore vision in patients. Retinal tear occur in patients when there is traction on the retina by the vitreous gel inside the eye while retinal detachment is caused by the breaking of sensory layer of retina allowing the fluid to seep underneath to detach the layer of retina. Retinal detachment is a serious disorder, which requires immediate treatment. (http://www.theretinasource.com/conditions/retinal_detachment.htm)

There are various methods used to treat retinal detachment, which include 1) Scleral Buckle, 2) Vitrectomy and 3) pneumatic retinopexy. One or combination of the above methods treat most retinal detachment disorders. In Scleral buckle, a silicone sponge or solid silicone is sewn to the Sclera, which is the outer wall of the eyeball, which pushes the retinal break and closes the break. The other two procedures either use

silicone oil in place of vitreous or gas bubble in the vitreous cavity to obtain the retinal attachment.
(http://www.vrmny.com/retinal_detachment.htm)

8.2.1 *Opthalmic implants*

A method of treatment is to culture glia cells on silicone foam, which is then implanted in the retina.   The material used is Poly-dimethyl-siloxane, which is selected for a high level of biocompatibility and non-toxicity and an ability to detach easily from the retina [Richter et al., 2000]. After the glia cell culture is merged with the retinal cells, the silicone foam is explanted (removed) and it is important that the foam does not adhere too strongly to the cells.

8.2.2 *Contact lenses*

Opthalmic devices and implants form an important division of external biomaterials. Myopia and hyperopia are the most common problems which many people currently face and use spectacles to correct the problems. Myopia referred to as short sightedness runs in to families in both elders and children due to different reasons. In this case the focus is obtained before reaching the macula in eye and the person has a blurred vision of distant objects. On the other hand in the case of hyperopia the patient suffers from far sightedness where the focus occurs after the macula for objects that are close to the eye. In both cases conventional treatment was to use the spectacles to correct this problem. Eyeglasses are useful in obtaining the correct focus of the object though it is an inconvenient method. Conventionally the eyeglasses were housed in plastic frames and sufficient care must be exercised to maintain them. However, with the advancements in medical science and materials it is now possible to get rid of the use of the eyeglasses. Contacts lenses have replaced the use of bulky uncomfortable eyeglasses for correction of Myopia/ Hyperopia in patients.
(http://www.eng.buffalo.edu/Courses/ce435/2001ZGu/Contact_Lens/ContactLensReport.htm)

Contact lenses are used by several millions of people, for reasons of either convenience or medical prescription. There are three basic types of contact lenses, the 'rigid gas permeable' contact lens, extended-wear (disposable) soft glass contact lens and the daily-wear soft glass contact lens.   The rigid gas permeable contact lens is made from transparent polymer typically obtained by copolymerizing methyl methacrylate (MMA) with methacrylo propyl trimethysilaxy silane (Tris) and allows atmospheric gases to diffuse through the lens. Contact lenses have improved the vision of users without subjecting them to risks of toxicity or allergy. The main problem with contact lenses is **keratitis**, which is infection and ulceration of the eyeball surface (*inflammation of cornea*) (http://www.youreyesite.com/kerartitis.htm).

In some cases, the severity of keratitis has been sufficient to cause near-blindness in the user [Cheng et al., 1999]. The moist conditions at the interface between the contact lens and the eyeball provide a fertile environment for pathogenic bacteria (e.g., pseudomonas aeruginosa and staphylococcus) and acanthamoebae [Cheng et al., 1999]. A practical solution to this problem is to avoid overnight wear of the lenses, which is considered to be a high-risk practice [Cheng et al., 1999]. The lowest risk of keratitis is associated with the use of rigid gas permeable contact lenses [Cheng et al., 1999]. The location of infection and mode of access by bacteria to the contact lens are illustrated schematically in Figure 8.1.

The annual incidence of keratitis (excluding mild cases which are unreported) ranges from approximately 1 incident per 10,000 users for rigid gas permeable lenses to approximately 20 per 10,000 users for extended wear soft lenses [Cheng et al., 1999]. The annual incidence of keratitis varies between countries because of different cleaning techniques and the precise value is a function of the study method [Cheng et al., 1999, Seal, 2000]. Correct cleaning procedures using proprietary cleaning fluids are found to be important [Seal, 2000].

Even with added disinfectants (chlorine tablets), tap water is found to be unsuitable because of contamination by acanthamoebae [Seal, 2000]. Rigid gas permeable contact lenses also display a poor adhesion characteristic to acanthamoebae, thereby facilitating cleaning and hindering infection. This is a significant advantage even if acanthamoebae cause only a minority of infections.

Other typical problems associated with contact lens include: Conjuctivitis epithelial microcyst, corneal edema, corneal neovascular-ization, Decompression sickness under a contact lens in conjunction with diving and infection [http://www.emedicine.com/EMERG/topic154.htm].

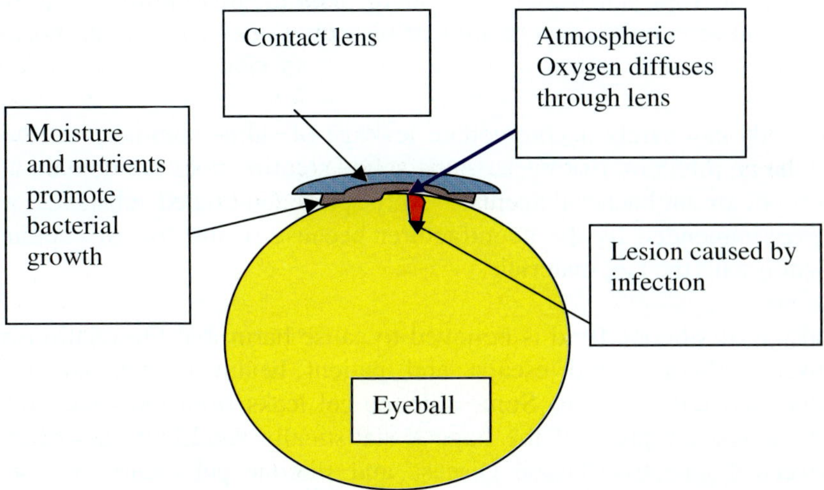

Fig 8.1. Infection of eyeball of wear of contact lenses.

8.3   Breast implants and IUD's

Breast implants and intrauterine devices share the feature of being exclusively fitted to ladies where they present some unique biomaterials problems.

8.3.1   *Breast implants*

Breast-implants are widely used for the restoration of form to female breasts. The implants consist of a fluid-filled flexible bag, which is placed by the surgeon under the mammary tissue or under the pectoral muscle. The bag is made of silicone, while the fluid may be either silicone gel or saline solution.

The surgical procedure is considered safe but not without risks of complications such as infection. Surgical revision to correct problems such as hard tissue formation around the implant or leakage is common. Breast implants are not expected to last for the lifetime of the patient [U.S.A, Food and Drug Administration (FDA)], the most common mode of failure is rupture of the implant and leakage of the fluid. Rupture of the bag is usually caused by excessive force on the breast (accidental impact), or from penetration by a sharp instrument. Rupture of the bag may occur after only a few months of service or after 10 years or more of service.

The body can safely accommodate leakage of saline solution, but there may be an infection risk because the saline solution does not contain any antiseptic or antibacterial agents.   Antiseptics and related substances are not recommended by the manufacturer because of the risk of chemical reaction with the bag material.

Leakage of silicone fluid is believed to cause harm, but the relationship between silicone fluid escape and patient health is still not fully understood [USA, FDA]. Some silicone gel leaks from most bags even without gross rupture of the bag. A statistically significant association between Connective Tissue Disease and silicone gel escape has been observed, but no significant association was observed with other auto-immune diseases such as rheumatism [USA, FDA].

One type of breast-implant was constructed of polyurethane foam, which released 2,4, toluenediamine (TDA) during service. It was found from urine analyses of implanted women, that the level of TDA release was too small to pose a significant health risk.   The manufacturer discontinued sales of this type of breast implant in 1991 [USA, FDA]. Chemical degradation studies of polyurethanes revealed that significant decay and release of TDA occurred only at temperatures in excess of 100 degrees Celsius or in severely alkaline conditions when tested at 37 degrees Celsius [Gott, 1997]. It was also found that TDA is rapidly excreted in the urine and faeces of patients [Gott, 1997], thus reducing the level of TDA exposure.   However, a long-term carcinogenic risk from TDA could not be entirely discounted [Gott, 1997].

8.3.2 *Intra-uterine devices*

The main risk with these devices appears to be the risk of severe infection and long-term damage to the reproductive system However, some corrosion of the metal parts of IUD's was observed [Chesney, 2000]. Despite the location of the IUD inside the female body, the IUD is not in intimate contact with vascular tissue (blood vessels).   This facilitates the selection of biomaterials, although it is still important to be stringently careful about issues such as contact sensitization.

8.4 Skin grafts

Skin grafts are widely used to restore skin on severely burnt patients. An earlier technique was to transplant skin from unburnt parts of the body to the burned part. The grafted skin would then grow to cover the surface of the body. A newer technique is to use a biodegradable polymer film, which acts as a substrate for the cultured growth of keratinocytes and dermal fibroblasts. Major problems with the polymer film are poor mechanical strength and immune rejection [Ng et al., 2000]. It is found that Poly (ε-Caprolactone) films provided a superior site for the growth of fibroblasts and keratinocytes into a cellular structure that is similar to that found in the human body [Ng et al., 2000]. An alternative material is polyurethane but this is observed to have inferior cell growth characteristics [Ng et al., 2000].

8.5 Materials for wound dressing

The natural healing of a wound is enhanced by a dressing, which inhibits further bleeding and helps to maintain good hygiene around the wound. Traditional dressings have been made from cotton sheets and gauze. There is now a greater range of dressings available [Heenan, 1998], the basic categories of dressing are listed below:

Synthetic fibre dressings
Polyurethane foam dressings
Alginate dressings (seaweed extract)
Cloth impregnated with activated charcoal and silver
Hydrocolloid dressings
Hydrogel dressings

The choice of dressing is largely based on how much liquid the wound is exuding and whether it is infected, not infected or necrotic (full of dead tissue) [Heenan, 1998].

8.5.1 *Synthetic fibre and polyurethane foam dressings*

Synthetic fibres have been increasingly used to replace the traditional cotton to make bandages and gauze. The main advantage of synthetic fibres over cotton is a reduced adhesion to the wound surface. Strong adhesion of a bandage to a wound can cause re-opening of the wound when the bandage is removed.

Polyurethane foam is used when the wound exudes a moderate amount of pus or other liquids.

8.5.2   *Alginate, hydrogel dressings*

These dressings differ fundamentally from the cotton and synthetic fibre dressings since they are water-soluble and can be washed off after healing of the wound. Alginates are derived from seaweed and can be formed into sheets or fibres. Alginate dressings consist of a hydrophilic gel and are very useful for absorbing liquids from heavily exuding wounds. Alginate dressings are however unsuitable for infected wounds. Allergic or inflammatory reactions to alginate dressings are rare, although some cases were recorded where a dressing was left in a wound for a long period of time. Chitin films are a promising form of treatment, with no apparent toxicity towards fibroblasts in the skin, no allergic response and only a moderate level of inflammation in the wound [Nealda et al., 2003].   The chitin films are formed from a 0.5% chitin solution where chitin flakes are dissolved in 5% solution of Lithium Chloride and N,N-dimethylacetamide. The chitin solution is poured into moulds where the chitin films form as a gel that is later cut out and pressed before use as a dressing. Tests on model cut wounds on rats revealed that the chitin films were effective as a dressing. Varying the density of water in the chitin film can be used to control the level of permeability to water of the chitin film. Reduced concentrations of water in the chitin film cause tighter bonding of the chitin molecular chains and lower permeability. A high permeability is suitable for wounds with a high level of exudates while drier wounds require a lower level of permeability to prevent the wound from drying out [Nealda et al., 2003].

Hydrogel dressings are used for the healing of dry or slightly exuding wounds only.   Some dry wounds may shed scabs and other layers of dead tissue or contain dead tissue (necrotic wounds). This dressing requires an outer layer of cloth to give mechanical stability. Hydrogel dressings are not suitable for infected wounds unless used in conjunction with maggot treatment.

8.5.3   *Cloth impregnated with activated charcoal and silver*

This dressing uses the properties of activated charcoal to absorb substances, which might facilitate bacterial growth. Silver is known to inhibit bacteria, so it is also included in the dressing. This type of dressing is useful for infected wounds.

8.5.4 *Hydrocolloid dressings and the maggot treatment of wounds*

Hydrocolloid dressings are one of the earliest types of non-traditional dressing and are widely used in modern medicine. The active ingredient of the hydrocolloid dressing is a hydrophilic (water absorbing) gel. Cellulose derivatives such as sodium carboxymethylcellulose and animal-derived subtances such as gelatin are used as gel-forming agents. The gel-forming agent is mixed with elastomers and adhesives and deposited on a thin polymer film.

Hydrocolloid dressings provide a moist environment to facilitate wound healing. It is found that hydrocolloid dressings with an appropriate outer covering of fine cloth provide a suitable medium for maggot treatment of wounds where the hydrocolloid is permeable to atmospheric oxygen, which the maggots require. The hydrocolloid is sufficiently flexible to allow the maggots to move freely and reach all the necrotic tissue present. Maggots of certain species of flies have been used for many centuries to remove (debride) dead and infected tissue from wounds [Kinshaw, 2000]. This allows the wounds to heal effectively without secondary infections, which might otherwise kill the patient. Only sterile maggots of fly species that do not attack living flesh are used, preferred fly species are the green and black bluebottles. Other fly species such as screwworm and Sarcophagidae (flesh flies) are unsuitable for this purpose because of their propensity for living flesh. The maggots (larvae of flies) consume the necrotic tissue in the wound and prevent bacteria from establishing colonies in the wound. It is believed that the mechanical disturbance of the maggots and their own secretions of digestive fluid prevent bacterial growth. With the increasing occurrence of antibiotic-resistant microbes, maggot treatment is regaining importance in the treatment of severe or chronic wounds. Hydrocolloid dressings and maggots are used for wounds, which have failed to heal after treatment with all known antibiotics.

Hydrocolloid dressings are not associated with allergic contact dermatitis (a common problem with dressings), but some forms of hydrocolloid may contain additives that generate adverse effects. A tackiness additive, pentaerythritol ester, is associated with sensitisation (initiation of allergy)

[Sasseville et al.,1997]. Tackiness is the property of adhesion to a wet surface and is a valued characteristic of hydrocolloid dressings.

8.6 Implants for cosmetic advantage

Developments in biocompatible and biodegradable implants have led to their potential use for cosmetic advantage. Typically these include facelift or enhancing appearance of other parts of the body such as breasts, abdomen etc. The breast implants have been dealt earlier in this chapter falls under this category. Typically facial implants used for face-lift (cosmetic advantage) are Gore-Tex (FDA approved materials), polypropylene, Teflon^{TM}, porous polyethylene and solid silicone. None of these materials are known to produce any adverse reactions. One of the problems associated with solid silicone is the migration of the implant. However, it is usually rare and use of porous polyethylene in place of silicone helps to avoid this problem by allowing tissue in growth and staying in position. Solid silicone is cheaper and is easily available compared to porous polyethylene. Other materials used for implants for facial lifts include metals such as cobalt chromium, stainless steel or titanium. Besides this hydroxyapatite is also used as implants for cheek, malar and sub malar plastic surgery. One of the typical disadvantages of these alloplastic implants is susceptibility for infection, which depends on various factors such as vascularity and positioning. (http://www.oralfacialsurgery.com/Cosmetics/
http://www.phudson.com/,http://www.drkorpeck.com/,).

8.7 Summary

Besides restoring functionality or repair of a damaged organ biomaterials are also used for cosmetic advantage. They can be either used externally to restore certain functions or protect the skin against infection such as contact lens and skin grafts respectively or used as an incision to improve the appearance. Opthalmic implants and contact lenses form an important category of biomaterials used either externally or mounted on the exterior of the body. Various materials are used for contact lenses such as PMMA, TRIS and similar polymers. The extended use of contact lens has certain disadvantages such as infections and protein deposition. Materials for wound dressings are a specialized form of external biomaterials, where the biomaterial characteristics are important for successful healing of the wound.

References

K.H. Cheng, S.L. Leung, H.W. Hoekman, W. Houdijn Beekhuis, P.G.H. Mulder, A.J.M. Geerards and A. Kijlstra, Incidence of contact-lens-associated microbial keratitis and its related morbidity, The Lancet, 1999, Vol. 354, No. 9174, 17 July 1999.

P.Joan Chesney, Infections of the female genital tract, *in* Infections Associated with Indwelling Medical Devices, 3rd edition, editors F.A. Waldvogel and A.L. Bisno, 2000, American Society of Microbiology Press, Washington, USA.

David Gott, Biodegradation and toxicokinetic studies, Chapter 3, in 'Biocompatibility Assessment of Medical Devices and Materials, editor, Julian H Braybrook, John Wiley and Sons, Chichester, United Kingdom, 1997, pp. 43-63.

Y. Haishima, T. Murai, Y. Nakagawa, M. Hirata, T. Yagami and A. Nakamura, Chemical and biological evaluation of endotoxin contamination on natural rubber latex products, Journal of Biomedical Materials Research, 2001, Vol. 55, No. 3, pp. 424-432.

A. Heenan, Dressings on the Drug Tariff, World Wide Wounds, 13 December 1998, edition 4.0

A. Heenan, Frequently asked questions: Alginate dressings, World Wide Wounds, 12 June, 1998, edition 1.0

A. Heenan, Frequently asked questions: Hydrocolloid dressings, World Wide Wounds, 28 April 1998, edition 1.1

J. Kinshaw, Larval therapy: a review of clinical human and veterinary studies, World Wide Wounds, October 2000, version 1.0

Marilynn Larkin, 'Latex allergy sparks new career, old fears', The Lancet, Vol.357, No. 9252, 27 January 2001.
www.thelancet.com/journal/vol357/iss9252/full/llan.357.9252.dissecting room.15020.1

Nealda L.B.M, A. Wee, Lee Y.L. and E. Khor, Flexible chitin films as potential wound-dressing materials: Wound model studies, Journal of Biomedical Materials Research Part, A, 2003, Vol. 66A, No. 2, pp. 224-232.

F.O. Nestle, H. Speidel and M.O. Speidel, High nickel release from 1- and 2- euro coins, Nature, 2002, Vol. 419, page 132.

K.W. Ng, S.H. Teoh, J.T. Schantz, D.W. Hutmacher, T.C. Lim, H.P. Too and T.T. Phan, A cell culture study on Poly (ε-Caprolactone) films, Proc. 10th International Conference on Biomedical Engineering, 6-9 December 2000, Singapore, edit. JCH Goh, publ. National University of Singapore, pp. 583-584.

H.A. Richter, M. Schmidbauer, H-Chr. Ludtke-Handjery and L. Hesse, 3D proliferation of glia cells in surface modified silicone foams as patch for retinal lesions, Proc. 10th International Conference on Biomedical Engineering, 6-9 December 2000, Singapore, edit. JCH Goh, publ. National University of Singapore, pp.130-131.

Sasseville D, Tennstedt D, Lachapelle JM: Allergic contact dermatitis from hydrocolloid dressings. American Journal of Contact Dermatitis1997 Dec;8(4):236-238

D.V. Seal, Contact-lens-associated microbial keratitis in the Netherlands and Scotland, The Lancet, 2000, Vol. 355, No. 9191, 08 January 2000.

http://www.emedicine.com/EMERG/topic154.htm

U.S. Food and Drug Administration, Centre for Devices and Radiological Health, Breast implants - an information update. http://www.fda.gov/cdrh/breastimplants

http://www.theretinasource.com/conditions/retinal_detachment.htm)
http://www.vrmny.com/retinal_detachment.htm
http://www.eng.buffalo.edu/Courses/ce435/2001ZGu/Contact_Lens/Cont actLensReport.htm
http://www.phudson.com/
http://www.drkorpeck.com/
http://www.oralfacialsurgery.com/Cosmetics/

Chapter 9

Tissue Scaffolds

9.1 Introduction

Tissue engineering is one of the recent developments in the field of biomaterials that has seen rapid progress over the past two decades. This technique is used for repair or regeneration of damaged tissues and organs to restore their functionality with the minimum surgical intervention. Tissue engineering involves the use of 'scaffolds' to facilitate growth of human cells. The prime motivation for the adoption of tissue scaffolds is a shortage of donor organs and the life-long administration of drugs to prevent immunorejection. Even if it is possible to avoid transplantation (which means sacrifice of tissue by another person) by the use of autografts, which is tissue from elsewhere in the patient's body, substantial problems remain. Second site morbidity of tissues and other patient associated problems (such as scarcity of suitable tissue) may occur. Tissue scaffolds are three-dimensional structures that are used for supporting the tissue or cells while the tissue regeneration or organ formation proceeds. The tissue scaffold can be classified according to the type of material used and the application. The scaffold is typically manufactured with a biodegradable polymer and provides usually (but not always) a temporary framework for the support of cells and the transport of nutrients to the tissues. The tissue and its cells are then expected to regenerate, thus allowing the scaffold to be safely discarded. Metallic materials have been used as scaffolds for the regeneration of hard tissue. One of the problems associated with metallic scaffolds is the stress shielding effect. This limitation is overcome by using polymeric scaffolds. Despite early success in developing scaffolds for tissue engineering, there are problems, which are yet to be resolved. In the case of biodegradable scaffolds, it is expected to decompose or resorb in the body after generation of the tissue/organ to restore functionality. Tissue scaffolds are gaining importance to re-grow articular cartilage and cardiac muscle, thus providing a cure for arthritis and heart disease. It is found that unless a suitable scaffold is present, specialized tissues such as cartilage and muscle cannot be restored.

Scaffolds, which are usually made from natural substances or from very benign hydrocarbons, are becoming recognized as a good substitute for metal prostheses. The construction and purpose of a scaffold is illustrated schematically in Figure 9.1.

A second more specialized type of scaffold is a drug release system, where particles or inclusions of pharmaceutical or antibody, are progressively released as the scaffold further degrades. This system allows the release of strong therapeutic agents at the site of the affected tissue, e.g., a tumour, with the minimum of detrimental effect to the overall health of the patient.

The mechanism of drug release by scaffolds is illustrated schematically in Figure 9.2.

The adoption of tissue scaffolds raises many new issues for service characteristics of materials. Whereas the conventional implant material should remain as inert as possible inside the body, the scaffolding material should respond to the metabolic processes of the body and display an affinity to human cells. Questions such as how quickly should the scaffold material degrade? Will the human cells adhere to the scaffold and remain viable? What is the effect of degradation on service performance e.g. is there a large increase in brittleness of the scaffold material? Are the degradation products harmful to the body? What is the maximum size of implant allowable before the rate of release of degradation products reaches a dangerous level? Questions like these, while not yet fully answered by current research, remain to be addressed by future researchers.

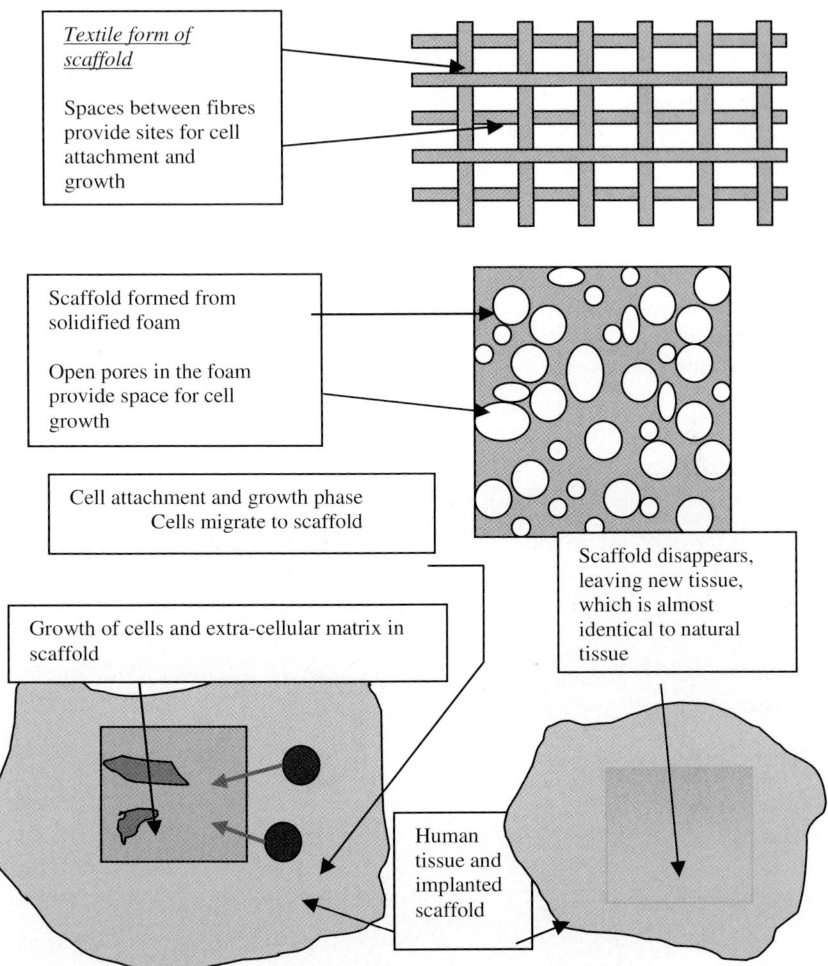

Fig 9.1. Construction and purpose of a scaffold.

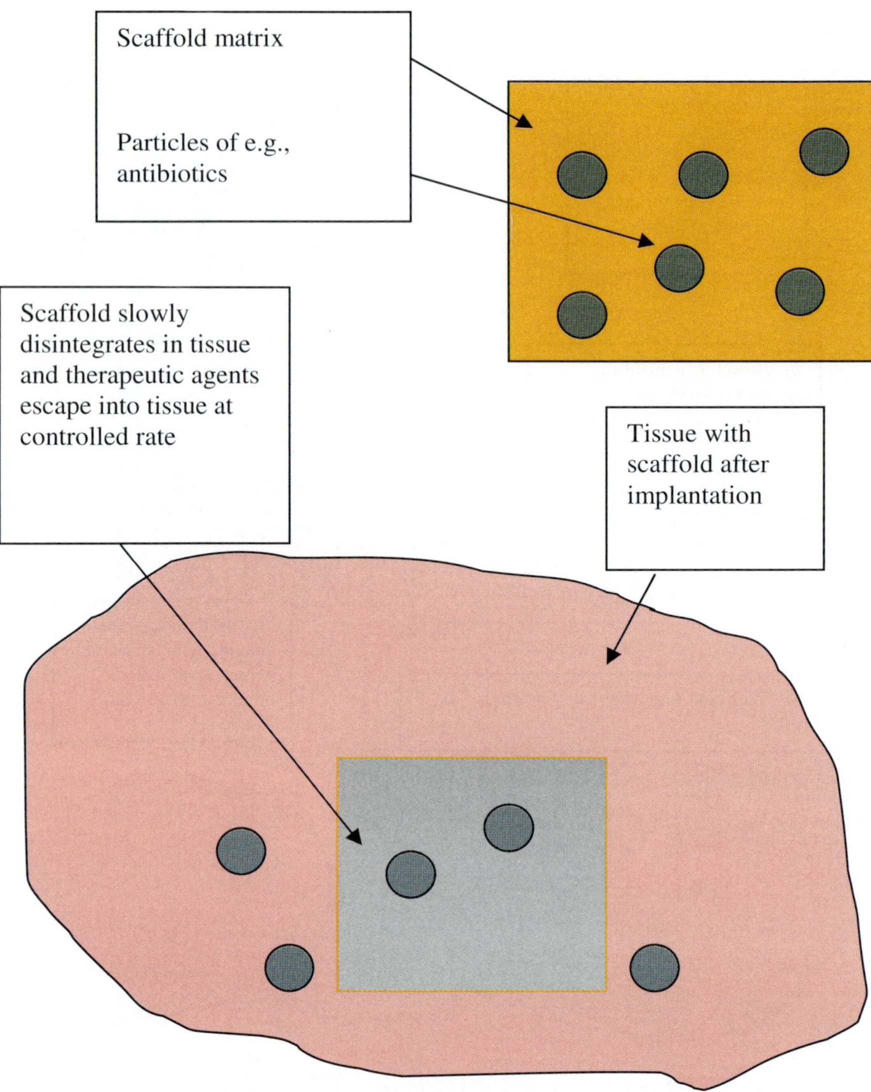

Fig 9.2. Localized drug delivery using a scaffold.

9.2 Biodegradable polymers and bioactive surfaces

One of the important requirements of a scaffold material is that the degradation products from the scaffold materials should be non-toxic. An important application of scaffold is the drug delivery system. Currently different types of materials are used for fabrication of a scaffold structure depending on the specific application. Polymers used for scaffolds can be broadly classified in to two group's namely natural and synthetic polymers. Collagen and Alginate fall under natural polymers while materials such as poly lactic acid or glycoloic acid and their derivatives, poly caprolactone etc., fall in to the category of synthetic biodegradable polymers. However, there are some concerns in the use of polymers with an acid or base group associated with them. Typically the degradation of these polymers releases the acid or base groups which change the local pH values. The change in local pH values affects the survival of the regenerated tissue thus defeating the purpose of scaffolding technique. A method to overcome this limitation is the use of bioresorbable materials, which tend to get resorbed in the body upon degradation without causing any adverse reactions. All the biodegradable polymers are designed to have a minimum strength during initial cell seeding and degrade with time while the damaged tissue or organ is regenerated. Almost all the biodegradable polymers undergo hydrolytic degradation in the presence of body fluids whose main constituent is water. The service lifetime, i.e. the period of time before bulk decomposition occurs, can be adjusted so that the tissue re-growth becomes sufficiently strong before the scaffold fails. Biodegradable polymers can be processed in different forms such as fibre, granules or foams. Fibres are used for creating a woven mesh with designated porosity and combination while foams are best applied in, as it is form in scaffolds. There are various techniques used for fabricating a three dimensional structure with desired porosity. Some of these techniques include solvent casting, particulate leaching, three-dimensional printing, fused deposition modeling etc. Though each of these techniques has the ability to produce scaffolds with different architecture, they have limitations with respect to various properties achievable. One of the important requirements of the scaffold is the highly interconnected pore network to facilitate transport of nutrients to the cell seeded. In particulate leaching, a poragen (generator of pores), i.e., sodium chloride, is added during manufacture of the scaffold. The sodium chloride is then removed by washing in water. Sodium chloride is chosen as the poragen because of its non-toxic characteristic. This technique produces pores of definite size depending on the size of the porogen used. One problem associated with this technique is the interconnectivity of pores, which cannot be controlled precisely. Techniques using rapid prototyping technology are able to produce definite architecture of porasity and interconnectivity. However, these techniques lack the strength requirements or use toxic organic solvents as binders, which limit their application. Techniques for the manufacture of scaffolds are rapidly advancing with 3-dimensional weaving of complex shapes that mimic parts of human organs [Landers and Mulhaupt, 2000].

Besides serving the function of a support structure a scaffold is also expected to have a certain amount of favourable environment for tissue ingrowth/ cell proliferation and differentiation. This function is served by inducing bioactivity to the surfaces of the scaffold. Here the term bio- activity refers to osteo induction/conduction. One example of induction of bioactivity is the use of hydroxyapatite coatings on ortheopedic protheses. Since hydroxyapatite, a synthetic ceramic, possesses a structure that resembles the organoapatite; the cells are able to attach to the apatite coating. Besides hydroxyapatite, various other materials such as biocompatible glasses are also used for inducing bioactivity.

Bioactive surfaces are surfaces designed to bond and merge with human cells. The most common application of bioactive surfaces is the hydroxyapatite coatings used in orthopaedic and dental applications. Bioactivity is a quality shared by a few materials for specific cell types. Most surfaces of artificial materials are not bioactive and have poor adhesion with cells.

9.3 Synthetic extra-cellular matrices

The human body contains many extra-cellular matrices, bone and cartilage being among the best examples. Where an extra-cellular matrix has been lost through injury or disease, a synthetic extra-cellular matrix may be used. Many scaffolds under development are intended as a temporary form of extra-cellular matrix, with material characteristics ranging from very strong to very pliable depending on the tissue application. Examples of very strong scaffolds are found in orthopaedic applications involving bone regrowth and more pliable scaffolds would be required for e.g., muscle regrowth (as in cardiac muscle).

9.3.1 *Scaffolding materials*

There are a wide variety of materials being tested for scaffolds but poly-ε-caprolactones and polylactides are frequently studied materials. Poly-dimethylacrylamide, polymethylmethacrylate, poly (lactic acid-glycolic acid) and polyurethanes have also been studied. Most of these polymers are used as fibres to form a woven fabric, which then serves as a scaffold. Another type of scaffold is based on foam, i.e. a highly porous solid, where the pores are typically a few tens of micrometres in average diameter. These foams are typically constructed of bioactive glass or calcium hydroxyapatite blends are intended for bone restoration. Chitosan, especially when blended with hydroxyapatites has also been studied as a scaffold material.

9.4 Applications of tissue scaffolds

There are two basic applications of scaffolds; (a) restoration of tissues using the scaffold as a template for human cells to attach and grow, (b) controlled and localized drug release for e.g., treating tumours, based on the slow escape of pharmaceutical compounds from a progressively disintegrating scaffold.

9.4.1 *Tissue engineering with scaffolds*

Currently, the main applications of tissue scaffolds are orthopaedic, cardiac and neural. All these applications involve the restoration of tissue composed of highly specialized cells and extra-cellular matrices.

Orthopaedic applications of tissue scaffolds involve the implantation of a block of scaffold material into a hole where arthritic cartilage has been removed. When the cartilage cells have grown to maturity within the scaffold, the cartilage is restored for sliding contact. Another orthopaedic application of tissue scaffolds is the restoration of bone that has been lost due to tissue inflammation from an implant failure. In this application, a scaffold formed from a bioactive glass, which is a blend of glass and apatite, was formed into a porous mass. Bone formation cells, i.e., osteo-progenitor cells, were then embedded in the pores for future integration with the glass [Livingston et al. 2002].

For the treatment of cardiac disease, the immediate objective is to develop the ability to grow patches of heart muscle, which can then be grafted to the weakened area of the patient's heart. For the treatment of neural problems, a tubular scaffold facilitates the re-growth of severed nerve fibres (see also chapter on cardiac and neural implants). This provides a treatment for paralysis caused after a fall or other impact.

An important application of tissue scaffold is in the maxillo facial/cranio facial reconstruction. Research indicates that almost US$3.5 billion is spent annually on maxillo-facial and cranio-facial surgery. Currently, titanium meshes are used for the cranio-facial and maxilla-facial surgery because of the mechanical strength and biocompatibility of titanium. However, researchers around the world are investigating the use of polymeric scaffolds for such reconstructions. The use of polymeric scaffolds for the reconstruction is being considered and suitable materials and various researchers around the world are investigating methods.

9.4.2 *Controlled and localized release of drugs*

Scaffolds based on poly (ε-caprolactone), poly (dimethylacrylamide), poly methylmethacrylate and other related co-polymers have been studied as materials for short-life time scaffolds. These materials were found to exhibit the required high levels of hydrophilicity (attraction to water), swelling and disintegration in the presence of water [Abraham et al., 2003]. It was found from an *in vivo* study (on pigs) that an inhibitor of glioma (a form of cancer) was almost entirely released from the scaffold 2 months after implantation.

Not all scaffold materials are designed to degrade within a period of 2 months or 60 days. Biodegradable polyurethanes constructed from poly (ε-caprolactone) diol, polyethylene oxide and other compounds were found to disintegrate significantly only after 48 weeks exposure in phosphate buffer solution [Gorna and Gogolewski, 2002]. For periods shorter than 2 months, a chitosan scaffold reinforced with calcium phosphate was found to offer sustained drug release for a period of 3 weeks. This composite is interesting since it can serve both as a drug release system and as a scaffold for the regeneration of bone [Zhang and Zhang, Vol. 62, 2002].

9.5 Three dimensional cell culture and the manufacture of scaffolds

9.5.1 *Manufacture of a the scaffold with a 3-dimensional structure*

In many cases, especially for the larger size of implants, a 3-dimensional structure is required for the scaffold. This presents a considerable challenge to engineering, with many radical new methods proposed. A recently developed method involves the use of a moving ultraviolet light pen that is controlled by a computer program. The ultra-violet light acts as an initiator of polymerization of a resin to allow construction of a structure in a step-wise manner [Matsuda and Mizutani, 2002]. In this case, the 3-dimensional structure is built layer by layer.

A major concern in the development of a large size scaffold is the facilitation of penetration of the scaffold by capillaries and larger blood vessels. This is especially important for the repair of ischaemic tissues (e.g., ischaemic heart muscle) and the development of organ replacements [Peters et al. 2002]. The fibres or surface of the scaffold can be coated with a vascular endothelial growth factor (VEGF) to encourage the growth of microvascular endothelial cells that have been transplanted into the scaffold.

9.5.2 *Manufacturing of precursors*

Scaffolds require specialized precursor materials; fine fibres composed of more than one organic polymer are commonly used. Electro-static spinning has been used to generate extremely fine fibres with diameter ranging from 0.5 to 0.8 micrometres in diameter [Li et al., 2002]. Electro-static spinning is a newly developed specialized process that is described below.

9.5.3 *Electrostatic spinning and the manufacture of extremely fine polymer fibres*

Conventional extrusion technology can only produce fibers with a diameter not less than 10 to 100 micrometres. Scaffolds and other textile implants often require a considerably smaller diameter of fibre. The manufacture of polymer fibres involves the extrusion of a semi-liquid jet when then solidifies to form a filament. When the diameter of the jet is less than a critical value, surface tension forces become strong enough to convert the jet into a series of droplets. If the liquid jet is however raised to a high electrical voltage, electro-static forces balance the surface tension and the jet remains largely undisturbed. This electro-static stabilization process is not perfect and beyond a certain distance, the jet still reverts to instability. However the distance of stable jet flow is long enough to allow useful manufacture of fibres. The electro-static spinning process was initially proposed almost 70 years ago but has only recently achieved prominence [Rutledge et al., 2001]. The process of electro-spinning as compared to conventional spinning is illustrated schematically in Figure 9.3. Voltages of 10's of kV are used for a free jet length of some 100's of mm, where the tested fibre materials include polycaprolactone and polyacrylonitrile. The electric current consumption is small, being measured in microamperes; hence the power consumption is also moderate. The electro-static spinning process enabled the success production of fibres as fine as 1 micrometre [Rutledge et al., 2001].

9.5.4 *Generation of porosity in scaffolding fibres*

The fibres used to construct a polymer scaffold should be porous to facilitate attachment and subsequent growth of cells. A recently proposed method of generating pores of close to the optimum number and size is based on co-extrusion. Two polymers, a water-insoluble polymer and a water-soluble polymer are blended together and co-extruded to form a composite material. Subsequent washing with water to remove the soluble polymer, allows the formation of pores with a controlled size in the polymer fibres. The elastic modulus of the porous material is also extremely low, approximately 1 MPa, to generate sufficient flexibility for the scaffold [Washburn et al.,2002]. A further advantage is that harmful solvents are not required to generate pores in the scaffold polymer. Considerable care is required to ensure that the scaffold does not contain even small amounts of toxic or carcinogenic substances.

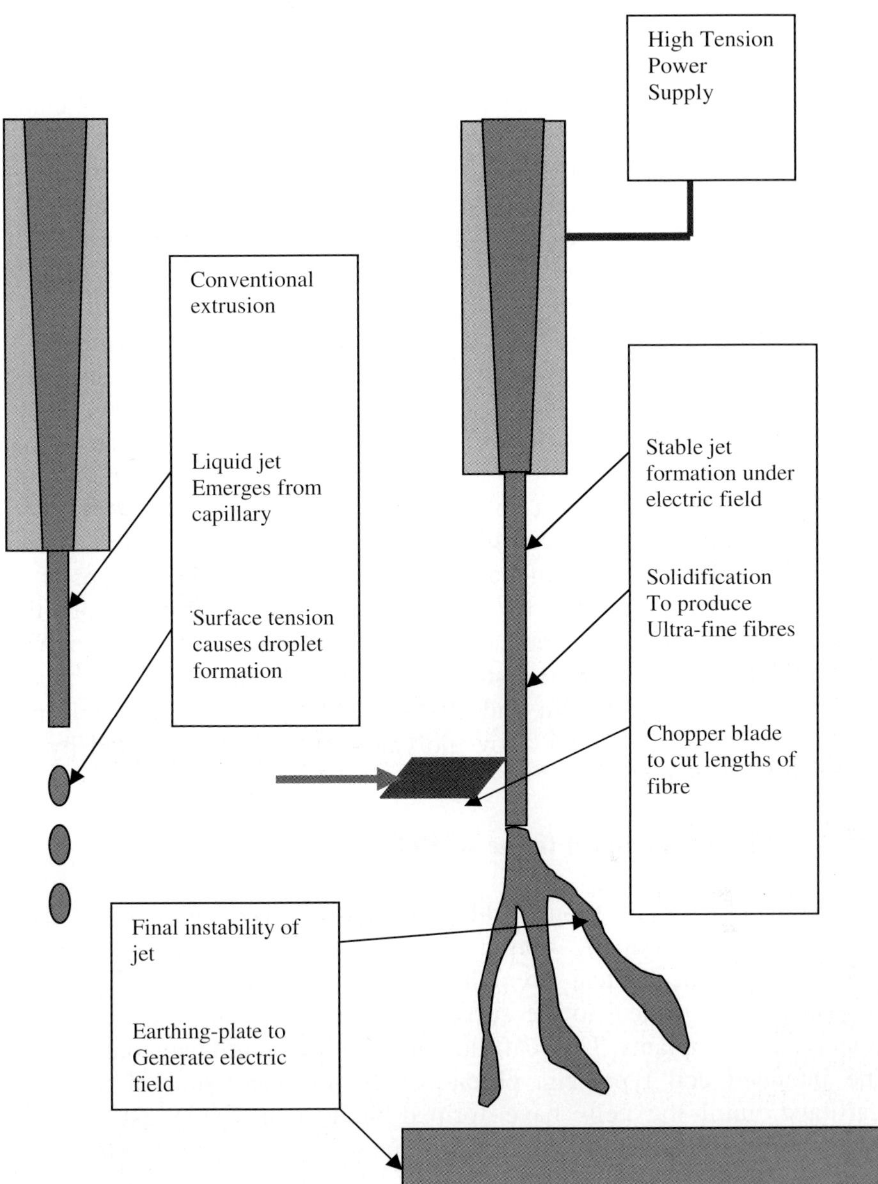

Fig 9.3. The principle of electrostatic spinning of ultra-fine fibres.

9.5.5 *Hydrogel scaffolds*

An alternative to the fibre-based scaffolds is the hydrogel scaffold. hydrogel is composed of water trapped by a network of long chain molecules. This forms a soft, moist solid that is similar to many forms of human tissue, e.g., cartilage. A blend of lysine and valine peptides (lysine and valine are amino acids) has been observed to form a hydrogel at concentrations as low as 2.0% [Henry, 2002]. The bulk constituent of the hydrogel, i.e. water, may enable delivery of water-soluble pharmaceuticals to adjacent tissue after implantation. Critical features of hydrogels are the use of natural amino acids that are enzymatically degradable to produce non-toxic decomposition products. The structure of the peptides should also be sufficiently ordered to prevent the formation of micelles. Micelles are spherical or spheroidal entities where water is enclosed by a shell of long-chain molecules. The micelles are usually too small to form a solid gel. Polyethylene oxide (PEO) and Polyvinyl alcohol (PVA) are used to form structural hydrogels that can facilitate the regeneration of natural cartilage. The basic concept is to inject an aqueous solution of precursor e.g., ethylene oxide into the human tissue. Once the aqueous solution is in place, polymerization is then initiated by light from a strong light source directed at the tissue [Paige et al., 1995; Anseth and Bryant , 2001]. Human tissue is not opaque to light and would allow polymerization to be initiated by an external light source.

9.6 Service problems of tissue scaffolds

Service problems of tissue scaffolds involve size limitations, toxic decomposition products, optimum mechanical strength and service period of the mechanical strength, affinity to human cells. Affinity to human cells is critical to the success of scaffolds, unlike conventional materials for implants. The scaffold must remain in intimate contact with the intended cell type, e.g. chrondocytes for restoration of synovial cartilage, until the cells have formed their own viable extracellular matrix. Uncontrolled growth of the tissue implant beyond the envisaged size has also been cited as a problem. Most tissue scaffolds lack the means to supply nutrients to the cells contained within the scaffold and likewise to remove the cellular waste products. This limitation is the result of the lack of capillaries within a scaffold. Beyond a certain size of scaffold, cells tend to grow on the exterior of the scaffold but not penetrate the interior of the scaffold.

9.6.1 *Mechanical strength of scaffolds*

A scaffold should have a useful level of mechanical strength, particularly for bone restoration applications. Compressive stress is of particular concern, both uniform and variable compressive stress. Scaffolds are usually arranged to sustain only compressive loading, at least in the initial growth stages to prevent detachment from the tissue. The scaffold should be able to resist compressive stress and maintain adequate living space for the cells that are attached to the scaffold. Static uniform compression inhibits the growth of chondrocytes in collagen scaffolds but variable load compression increased the growth rate of chondrocytes [Lee et al., 2003]. The type of compressive loading, i.e. static or variable, also affects the distribution of cells in the scaffold structure. Static loading gives rise to a heterogeneous (non-uniform) cell distribution, while variable loading promotes a homogeneous cell distribution [Burg et al., 2002]. The difference in cell distribution and growth rates may be due to better flushing of nutrients through the scaffold by variable loading (with the resultant variable elastic deformation). The development of a strong load bearing structure in a scaffold requires a significant amount of time. A scaffold of porous bioactive glass was found to require 12 weeks of implantation before bone strength was restored. Tissue-engineering the same scaffold with osteo-progenitor ('bone-seeding') cells reduced the time required for bone regrowth to 4 weeks [Livingston et al., 2002].

Compressive modulus is an important service parameter of orthopaedic scaffolds; an advantage of incorporating bioactive glass into a polymer (polylactide-co-glycolide) scaffold is the increase in compressive modulus achieved. This is in addition to the enhancement of osteointegration that is provided by the bioactive glass [Lu et al., 2003].

9.6.2 *Service life of scaffolds*

The degradation rate of the scaffold is a critical performance characteristic. It is found that the persistence of residual scaffold material *in vivo* may be much longer than expected by *in vitro* tests. Specimens of poly-L-lactide placed in the cancellous bone of rabbits were found to persist at least as long as the 4.5 year duration of the experimental study [Laitinen et al., 2002].

Another in *vivo* study on polymer fibres implanted sub-cutaneously in rats, revealed that the response of the surrounding tissue is dependent on the diameter of the fibre. 1 – 5 micrometre diameter fibres of polyester, polyethylene, polylactic acid and polyurethane caused significantly less fibrous capsule formation than 11-15 micrometre diameter fibres of the same material [Sanders et al., 2002]. The response of the tissue to the scaffold is not entirely controlled by the scaffold material but is also influenced by the physical form of the material.

In most cases the decomposition products from the scaffold material are non-toxic; however there may be abnormally sensitive individuals among the patients. It is possible for the scaffold to be too successful, since the implanted tissue may continue to grow beyond its intended limits. This uncontrolled growth has been anecdotally likened to cancer.

9.6.3 *Promotion of cell growth inside the scaffold*

Rapid and effective attachment of cells to either the fibres or pores of a scaffold is a critical service characteristic. Surface coatings of amino acids and peptides within a porous poly(lactic acid) scaffold was observed to lead to more rapid growth of bone cells during *in vitro* tests [Hu et al., 2003]. A more radical approach involving anhydrous ammonia plasma treatment was found to improve the hydrophilic characteristics and surface energy of poly (L-lactic acid) and poly(L-lactic acid –co-glycolic acid) where the growth and retention of human fibroblast cells was enhanced [Yang et al., 2002].

Cell growth is also influenced by the physical characteristic of pore size, where a size range of 160 micrometres [Yang et al. 2002] for human skin fibroblasts and 100 micrometres for bone tissue [Zhang and Zhang, 2002, Vol. 61] are considered to the most favourable for cell growth.

9.7 Summary

Scaffolds represent the most recent change in service requirements of biomedical materials. The traditional biomaterial was formulated to maximize strength and inertness or at least only a controlled bioactivity. Some scaffolds are often made deliberately weak and pliable to minimize damage to tissues and have a pre-arranged finite service life, which is generally much shorter than the decades expected of e.g., orthopaedic implants. Other scaffolds however must still possess significant levels of mechanical strength, particularly compressive strength. Non-traditional service parameters such as hydrophilicity, resorption rate and release rate of entrained drugs are critically relevant to scaffold material performance.

References

G.A. Abraham, A. Gallardo, J.S. Roman, A. Fernandez-Mayoralas, M. Zurita and J. Vaquero, Polymeric matrices based on graft copolymers of PCL onto acrylic backbones for releasing anti-tumoral drugs, Journal of Biomedical Materials Research, 2003, Vol. 64A, pp. 638-647.

K.S. Anseth and S.J. Bryant, The effects of scaffold thickness on tissue engineered cartilage in photo-crosslinked poly(ethylene oxide) glycogels, Biomaterials, 2001, Vol. 22, pp. 619-626.

K.J.L. Burg, M. Delnomdedieu, R.J. Beiler, C.R. Culberson, K.G. Greene, C.R. Halberstadt, W. D. Holder Jr., A.B. Loebsack, W.D. Roland, G.A. Johnson, Application of magnetic resonance microscopy to tissue engineering: A polylactide model, Journal of Biomedical Materials Research, 2002, Vol. 61, No. 3, pp. 380-390.

K. Gorna and S. Gogolewski, Biodegradable polyurethanes for implants. II. *In vitro* degradation and calcificationof materials from poly (ε-caprolactone)-poly(ethylene oxide) diols and various chain extenders, Journal of Biomedical Materials and Materials Research, 2002, Vol. 60, No. 4, pp. 592-606.

C. Henry, Block polypeptide hydrogels, CENEAR (Chemical engineering News), 2002, Vol. 80, No. 21, page 14.

Y. Hu, S.R. Winn, I. Krajbich and J.O. Hollinger, Porous polymer scaffolds surface-modified with arginine-glycine-aspartic acid enhance bone cell attachment and differentiation *in vitro*, Journal of Biomedical Materials Research, 2003, Vol. 64A, No. 3, pp. 583-590.

O. Laitinen, H. Pihlajamaki, A. Sukura and O. Bostman, Transmission electron microscopic visualization of the degradation and phagocytosis of a poly-L-lactide screw in cancellous bone: A long-term experimental study, Journal of Biomedical Materials Research, 2002, Vol. 61, No. 1, pp. 33-39.

R. Landers and R. Mulhaupt, Complex objects and tailor-made scaffolds fabricated by means of three dimensional plotting of biodegradable thermoplastics, thermosets and hydrogels, Proc. 10th International Conference on Biomedical enginering, 6-9 December 2002, Singapore, edit. JCH Goh, publ. National University of Singapore, pp. 132-133.

C.R. Lee, A.J. Grodzinsky and M. Spector, Biosynthetic response of passaged chondrocytes in a type II collagen scaffold to mechanical compression, Journal of Biomedical Materials Research, 2003, Vol. 64A, pp. 560-569.

W.-J. Li, C.T. Laurencin, E.J. Caterson, R.S. Tuan and F.K. Ko, Electrospun nanofibrous structure: A novel scaffold for tissue engineering, Journal of Biomedical Materials Research, 2002, Vol. 60, No. 4, pp. 613-621.

T. Livingston, P. Ducheyne and J. Garino, *In vivo* evaluation of a bioactive scaffold for bone tissue engineering, Journal of Biomedical Materials Research, 2002, Vol. 62, No. 1, pp. 1-13.

H.H. Lu, S.F. El-Amin, K.D. Scott and C.T. Laurencin, Three-dimensional, bioactive, biodegradable, polymer-bioactive glass composite scaffolds with improved mechanical properties support collagen synthesis and mineralization of human osteoblast-like cells in vitro, Journal of Biomedical Materials Research, 2003, Vol. 64A, No. 3, pp. 465-474.

T. Matsuda and M. Mizutani, Liquid acrylate-endcapped biodegradable poly ε-caprolactone-*co*-trimethyl carbonate).I. Preparation and visible light-induced photocuring characteristics, Journal of Biomedical Materials Research, 2002, Vol. 62, No. 3, pp. 387-394.

T. Matsuda and M. Mizutani, Liquid acrylate-endcapped biodegradable poly ε-caprolactone-*co*-trimethyl carbonate). II computer-aided stereolithographic microarchitectural surface photoconstructs, Journal of Biomedical Materials Research, 2002, Vol. 62, No. 3, pp. 395-403.

K.T. Paige, L.G. Clima, M.J. Yaremchuk, J.P. Vacanti and C.A. Vacanti, Injectable Cartilage, Plastic and Reconstructive Surgery, 1995, Vol. 96, pp. 1390-1400.

M.C. Peters, P.J. Polverini and D.J. Mooney, Engineering vascular networks in porous polymer matrices, Journal of Biomedical Materials Research, 2002, Vol. 60, No. 4, pp. 668-678.

G.C. Rutledge, Y. Li, S. Fridrikh, S.B. Warner, V.E. Kalyci and P. Patra, Electrostatic spinning and properties of Ultrafine fibers, National Textile Center Annual Report: November 2001, M01-D22

J.E. Sanders, S.D. Bale and T. Neumann, Tissue response to microfibers of different polymers: Polyester, polyethylene, polylactic acid and polyurethane, Journal of Biomedical Materials Research, 2002, Vol. 62, No. 2, pp. 222-227.

P. Sepulveda, A.H. Bressiani, J.C. Bressiani, L. Meseguer and B. Konig, *In vivo* evaluation of hydroxyapatite foams, Journal of Biomedical Materials Research, 2002, Vol. 62, No. 4, pp. 587-592.

T. Taguchi, T. Ikoma and J. Tanaka, An improved method to prepare hyaluronic acid and type II collagen composite matrices, Journal of Biomedical Materials Research, 2002, Vol. 61, No. 2, pp. 330-336.

N.R. Washburn, C.G. Simon, A. Tona, H.M. Elgendy, A. Karim and E.J. Amis, Co-extrusion of biocompatible polymers for scaffolds with co-continuous morphology, Journal of Biomedical Materials Research, 2002, Vol. 60, No. 1, pp. 20-29.

J. Yang, G. Shi, J. Bei, S. Wang, Y. Cao, Q. Shang, G. Yang and W. Wang, Fabrication and surface modification of macroporous poly (L-lactic acid) and poly (L-lactic-*co*-glycolic acid) (70/30) cell scaffolds for human skin fibroblast cell culture, Journal of Biomedical Materials Research, 2002, Vol. 62, No. 3, pp. 438-446.

Y. Zhang and M. Zhang, Three-dimensional macroporous calcium phosphate bioceramics with nested chitosan sponges for load-bearing bone implants, Journal of Biomedical Materials Research, 2002, Vol. 61, No. 1, pp. 1-8.

Y. Zhang and M. Zhang, Calcium phosphate/chitosan composite scaffolds for controlled *in vitro* antibiotic drug release, Journal of Biomedical Materials Research, 2002, Vol. 62, No. 2, pp. 378-386.

Chapter 10

Physiological Reactions to External Support Systems

10.1 Introduction

Besides reactions of physiological medium with implant materials used in applications such as hip prostheses, heart valves or tissue scaffolds, the reactions and biocompatibility of external support systems play an important role. These can range from simple devices used for monitoring blood pressure to complex systems used for dialysis. The insertion of any device into the human body carries a risk of infection even though the basic purpose of the device may be medical treatment. An example of such problems is the urinary catheter, which is a common cause of urinary tract infections. A urinary catheter coated with gentamicin sulfate (an antiobiotic) has been developed in order to reduce the risk of infection [Kim et al., 2000]

10.2 Kidney dialysis

A major problem in kidney dialysis machines is the leaching of catalysts and stabilizers from the polymers used for tubing in the machine. The catalysts are often heavy metals, which are toxic. These polymerization agents enter the blood and are then conveyed to all parts of the patient's body by blood circulation. It is found that acute sclerosis of they eyes may occur as a result [Vienken,2000]. Blood is found to be a very active leaching medium of polymers because of its wide range of fats and proteins. It is very difficult to select a polymer of suitable mechanical properties that is resistant to leaching by blood [Vienken,2000]. The polymer tubing may also interact with medicinal drugs taken by patient with strong side effects such as a severe loss of blood pressure [Vienken,2000].

Sterilization of polymers for dialysis systems faces difficulties because of the low temperature limits of most polymers. This limits the maximum temperature in an autoclave. A common practice is to sterilize the polymer tubing with ethylene oxide, but it is necessary to remove all residual ethylene oxide from the tubing before use [Vienken,2000].

Protein absorption on the inner surfaces of the polymer tubing also requires control, because of mechanical blockage of the small diameter tubes and causes blood clotting or other physiological cascades [Vienken,2000].

The intense flow of blood through the fine tubing of a dialysis system can also cause loss of mechanical toughness in the polymer used to make the tubing. A progressive loss of ductility with duration of dialysis duty was found for cellulosic-based fibres used in Hemophan ME-10H type dialysers [Konduk and Ucisik]. Microscopic evidence of flow erosion or leaching by the dialysate was observed together with chemical changes evidenced by XRD (X-ray Diffractometry) and DSC (Differential Scanning Calorimetry).

Some (but not all) dialysis tubing is made of Polyvinyl chloride (PVC). PVC is very brittle and is commonly mixed with a type of phthalate, di-2-ethylhexyl-phthalate (DEHP) that acts as a plasticizer [Tickner et al., 2001]. Leaching of DEHP from the PVC tubing and into the body leads to its partial conversion to MEHP (mono-ethylhexyl-phalate). MEHP is associated with testicular and heart damage while DEHP mimics the action of the hormone oestrogen. The intense liquid flow within dialysis tubing is not essential for leaching of DEHP, this can occur in the quiescent environment of a blood bag or intravenous infusion bag [Tickner et al., 2001]. Tests of PVC outside of the medical context reveal how easily this compound is degraded to release chemically active products. Rolling contact under water irrigation between a steel rod and a PVC wheel was shown to cause release of chlorides [Hamblin and Stachowiak, 1995].

10.3   External blood pumps

Blood pumps range from remote systems that are connected to the body only by tubes and partially implanted systems where a pump is placed in the body but the power source remains outside of the body. The purpose of external blood pumps is to provide a substitute for the heart while it is incapacitated either by disease or during a surgical operation. The partially implanted heart pumps are used to provide short to medium term relief for patients who are awaiting a heart-transplant. A common design is the Left Ventricle Assist Device (LVAD), which is fitted inside the body with a shoulder mounted external power supply.

Blood pumps suffer from the same problems of haemolysis (damage to red blood cells) and clotting that occur in cardiac implants. Careful design of the pump is critical since pumps are associated with high flow velocities and shear rates, which can affect the cellular population of the blood. There is also a risk of infection from the implantation of the heart pump. In pumps tubing plays a vital role in carrying body fluids into the body. It also serves as a means to carry nutrients, electrolytes and drugs into the body, besides acting as a medium of extracorporeal circulation of blood during surgery. During this process the tubing should be strong enough with sufficient flexibility to maintain consistent flow through them and should not be distorted. Typically silicone elastomers are used for tubing applications in blood pumps and dialysis equipment due to their biocompatibility. These elastomers are either cured using two different methods namely peroxide curing and platinum curing. Peroxide cured silicone tubes withstand the stringent tests and possess the required physical properties for long-term stability but need to undergo a post cure step to remove toxic by-products generated while platinum curing has low levels of by-product generation. The platinum cured silicone elastomer tubes fail the rigorous tests for which certify its usage in external blood pumps [Baity, 1998].

Despite the biocompatibility of materials used in medical devices that are blood contacting, the finished product may not possess the same level of biocompatibility due to factors such as geometry or processing methodology altering the surface chemistry of the material. Hence the medical devices used can cause clotting of blood thereby impairing the functionality of such devices. One of the methodologies currently adopted is to use hemocompatible material coatings on the tubing to overcome blood clotting.   Heparin is widely used for obtaining a hemocompatible coating on tubing. However another method is to use a bioinert material instead of heparin so that the blood does not respond to the presence of a foreign body during circulation. Besides serving the purpose of improving the hemocompatibility, coatings may be designed to provide the lubricity with antimicrobial properties. Such coatings may not only serve to improve the hemocompatibility but also kill the bacteria that may cause thrombus formation in blood [Spice,2001].

10.4   Ventricular assist devices and monitoring

Variety of mechanical devices has been designed for problems associated with heart failure, which we have seen in chapter 5. However the use of implantable ventricular assist devices typically serves as a bridge to transplantation, which is the only available solution for heart failure. Typically most VAD's are not suitable for long-term usage due to the problems associated with thromboembolism caused by direct blood contact with the pumping chamber. A possible solution is the use of electromechanically actuated woven fiber to pump the heart. The mechanical device does not need to perform the function of the heart and serves as a support for the heart with an auxiliary source of mechanical power.

Another typical external support device is the use of mechanical ventilators for forcing oxygen into the lungs. But a serious limitation of such breathing devices is that it cannot be used when the lungs itself is damaged. Patients with damaged lungs need to undergo a lung transplant. To keep the patient alive until a suitable donor is available. The heart lung machines that are used during heart surgery are candidates for artificial lungs. But these are expensive and are prone to complications and thus limit their usage. Dr. Brack Hattler developed a short-term lung assist device, which can add oxygen to blood and remove carbon dioxide. The device is known as hattler respiratory catheter, which is inserted to large vein carrying blood back to the heart. This device is typically useful in patients who have had injury or acute disease and lungs are recovering.

10.5 Summary

This chapter deals with the external support systems commonly used in medicine. The toxicity caused due to leaching during dialysis and external blood pumps. Functional requirements of mechanical ventilators and catheter tubes and modifications required to avoid thrombosis of blood in the catheter has been explained.

References

M.G. Hamblin and G.W. Stachowiak, Environmental and sheave material effects on the wear of roping wire and sheave, Tribology International, 1995, Vol. 28, No. 5, pp. 307-315.

S.H. Kim, K.B. Lee, J.M. Choi, Y.H. Cho, Y.H. Bae, S.Y. Jeong and I.C. Kwon, Preparation of Gentamicin-releasing urethral catheter for short-term catheterization, Proc. 10th International Conference on Biomedical Engineering, 6-9 December 2000, Singapore, edit. JCH Goh, publ. National University of Singapore, pp.379-380.

B.A. Konduk, A.H. Ucisik, Comparative changes in mechanical behavior of polymeric fibers used in hemodialysis, , Proc. 10th International Conference on Biomedical Engineering, 6-9 December 2000, Singapore, edit. JCH Goh, publ. National University of Singapore, pp. 507-508.

Bryon Spice, Pitt at work on 2 kinds of breathing machines Thursday, April 26, 2001 By Byron Spice, Science Editor, Post-Gazette.

Joel A. Tickner, Ted Schettler, Tee Guidotti, Michael McCally and Mark Rossi, Health Risks posed by use of Di-2-ethylhexyl phthalate (DEHP) in medical devices, American Journal of Industrial Medicine, 2001, Vol. 39, No.1, pp. 100-111.

Jorg Vienken, Polymers in Nephrology, needs, properties and performance, Proc. 10th International Conference on Biomedical Engineering, 6-9 December 2000, Singapore, editor. JCH Goh, publ. National University of Singapore.

Medical Device & Diagnostic Industry <u>Magazine</u> <u>MDDI Article Index</u> An MD&DI January 1998 Column Tubing Applications Characterizing Silicone Elastomers for Pump Tubing Applications, Judith Fairclough Baity.

Coatings Hemocompatible Coatings for Blood-Contacting Devices Coating makers take many different paths to ensure the blood compatibility of medical products. Originally Published <u>MDDI</u> August 2003 William Leventon.

Chapter 11

Drug Delivery Systems

11.1   Introduction

Drug delivery systems have traditionally involved a pill, a skin patch, an inhaler or an injection. All of these methods suffer from limitations in controlling the dosage rate and drug distribution of the therapeutic substance all over the body instead of to the diseased or weakened tissue site. For example, the ingestion of oral drugs is associated with a sharp rise in blood concentrations of the drug followed by a gradual decline in concentration. Malignant tumors can be effectively treated by high, localized concentrations of radioactive elements that are harmful to normal tissue. Recently there is a rapid development in the encapsulation of the therapeutic substances that will mitigate these problems. Any safe technology that offers effective therapy to the patient is tried. For instance, a treatment for retinal vein blockage involves a fine probe, which releases a small electric discharge to vapourize a saline solution of plasminogen. The vigorous flow of fluid during vapourization delivers the plasminogen to the blockage inside the vein. It is hoped that this mode of treatment will help save the eyesight of many patients [Sample, 2001]. The new type of drug delivery systems involves encapsulating the therapeutic substance in an entity, which can be regarded in some cases as an advanced material or in other cases as a nano-system. In most instances, the drug encapsulation/carrier system is for single use only. The prime questions for these new drug delivery systems from the viewpoint of service characteristics include questions such as what durability is required of the delivery system. Does the delivery system safely degrade within the human body without releasing toxic substances? What characteristics of the material are required to ensure controlled drug delivery? How can the material be engineered to enable discrimination between different types of tissues?   These and other questions are briefly reviewed in this chapter along with some estimation of future advances in drug delivery systems. In this rapidly developing research topic, the discussion presented here must be provisional in nature.

Drug delivery can be broadly classified into two categories namely, controlled release of drug and targeted drug delivery. In case of targeted drug delivery system the drug is encapsulated and isolated. The encapsulation permits the diffusion or release of drug only to the specific organ, tissue or cell. This is normally achieved by designing a suitable encapsulation, which will release the drug only when certain environmental conditions are present within the body. The environment of interest can be local concentration of body fluids, pH value of the fluid or physiochemical properties of the polymeric matrix used as a drug carrier such as molecular weight, solubility of the polymer and glass transition temperatures etc. Controlled release of drug typically follows release patterns based on the diffusion kinetics. Sustained release drugs usually fall into this category of drug release where the kinetics follows either a first order equation or zero order equation. Typical patterns of zero and first order kinetics of drug delivery is depicted in Figure 11.1.

Fig 11.1. First order kinetics of drug release and Zero order kinetics of drug release Ref Biomedical Engineering Handbook.

A variety of parameters influence this type drug release such as device geometry (encapsulation geometry), the physiochemical properties of the polymer matrix in which the drug is loaded (molecular weight, crystallinity, glass transition temperatures etc), interaction between the drug and its matrix with associated osmotic pressures. The ideal expected release rate of drugs should follow zero order kinetics in order to have maximum effect with minimum side effects of the said drug. This type of release kinetics is normally achieved by encapsulation of the drug in a matrix that provides passive diffusion of the drug. During the period of drug release it is expected that the drug remains thermodynamically stable. The matrix usually consists of a non-degradable polymeric material. This type of drug release has a potential risk of drug overdose or blocking of supply of drug due to failure of the matrix or a change in physiochemical properties of the encapsulating polymer. The controlled release mechanism has been found to be ineffective in maximizing the drug interactions while minimizing the side effects of the drug in most cases due to varying nature of the environmental conditions present in the body. To have a maximum pharmacological effect, drug targeting on a specific organ, tissue or cell is preferred over controlled release rates of drugs.

11.2   Physicochemical and mass transfer considerations in microencapsulation

Micro-encapsulation has been widely used in polymeric drug delivery systems and cell therapy. Micro-encapsulation typically faces problems with the mass transfer across the encapsulation. The release of the bioactive agent (drug) from the encapsulation (polymer matrix/capsule) should involve a reliable mechanism for constant release of drug. A typical example is release of insulin in diabetes treatment, which diffuses out of the capsule along with low molecular weight waste products while supplying the necessary oxygen to the immobilized cells.

To gain a better understanding of the physicochemical and mass transfer in micro-encapsulation, the oxygen transport, mass transfer coefficients, concentration of the cell immobilization matrices, the loading of the microcapsule and the diffusivity of oxygen in the immobilization agent in the microcapsule should be analyzed in detail.

A typical example of mass transfer in the physicochemical context can be seen in cell transplantation/cell therapy for treatment of insulin dependent diabetes. Encapsulation used for cell therapy or drug delivery should ensure diffusion of nutrients and release of the drug. The mass transfer rate within the micro-encapsulation can be altered by varying the signals to the encapsulation such as change in pH, release of ions, temperature, electric current, photo irradiation, magnetic field and ultrasound. These signals modulate the diffusion rate of the drug thereby enabling a pulsatile release or a timed program release of drugs. To achieve such programmed drug release, it is essential to know the physicochemical properties of the polymer such as molecular weight, crystallinity, glass transition temperature, melting points, diffusivity, the degradation rate and any environmental effects (e.g. change in pressure for deep-sea divers). An external stimulus, which is either thermally activated or by other means, affects the degradation rate and the physicochemical properties of the polymer. This in turn alters the mass transport rates within the micro-encapsulation resulting in modulated drug release.

11.3   Materials for the selective delivery of drugs

Fullerenes are currently being studied as a means of delivering radioactive isotopes to malignant tumors without releasing these dangerous isotopes into healthy tissues [Vogelson, 2001]. Fullerenes consist of a circular cage of carbon atoms that can contain the metal radioisotope and resist enzymatic degradation inside the body. Experimental tests revealed that the Fullere-radioisotope system preferentially accesses bone tissue (for e.g., the treatment of leukemia) [Vogelson, 2001]

For selective delivery of drugs, non-degradable polymers are preferred over degradable polymers. Specific applications such as drug delivery for angiogenesis also use micro spheres derived from alginate beads or similar natural polymers. Some of the typical polymers used include polydimethylsiloxane (PDMS), polyurethanes (PU) and polyethelenecovinylacetate (EVAc copolymers). These polymers are attractive candidates for reservoir type drug delivery system, which are implantable for long-term applications. PU has been used in local delivery of cardiovascular drugs and for non-thrombogenic surfaces in cardiovascular implants. Other polymers that are used for controlled and selective delivery of drugs include poly (2-hydroxy ethylmethacrylate), a hydrogel used commonly in soft contact lens. These polymers are used in reservoir type drug delivery system with a predefined diffusion barrier to provide the necessary release rate of the drug. Stimuli sensitive polymeric materials, which are non-biodegradable, should be used for modulated or pulsatile drug delivery. A typical mechanism by which pulsatile drug release takes place is presented in Figure 11.2.

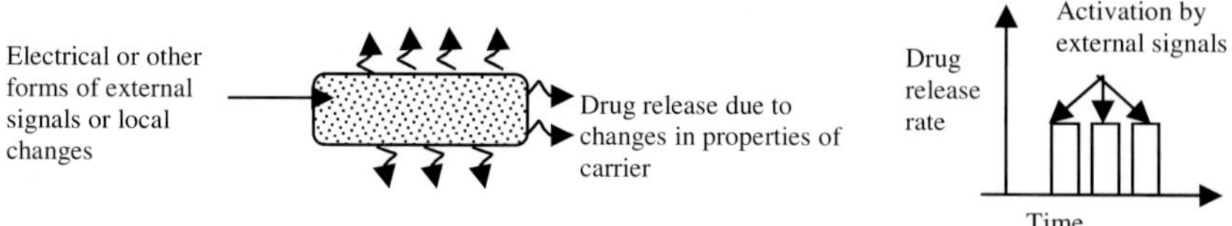

Fig 11.2. Mechanism of pulsatile release or time programmed release of drugs.

11.4 Materials for sustained release of drugs

Controlled release of insulin into the blood stream is vital for the effective management of diabetes. The insulin is contained in a hydrogel, which also contains an immobilized form of the enzyme, glucose oxidase. When there is an excess of sugar present in the blood, the enzyme (indirectly) converts glucose to gluconic acid, which lowers the pH (acidity) and stimulates the hydrogel to release insulin into the blood [Vogelson, 2001]. This system is still at the initial stages of development, a future question for service characteristics is how long would this system remain reliable? Ideally, the system should remain reliable until all the insulin contained in the hydrogel has been exhausted.

For controlled release both degradable and non-degradable polymers can be used. In this case, degradable polymers are high molecular weight substances, which encapsulate the drug and later decompose into non-toxic monomer. Biodegradable polymers are either synthetic or natural. Polymers of polysaccarides and proteins fall under the natural biodegradable polymers. The synthetic polymers consist of aliphatic polyesters of polylactide (PLA), polyglycolide, poly (lactide-co-glycolyde) and other polymers such as polycaprolactene (PCL) etc. The most widely used synthetic biodegradable polymer is PLA. Biodegradable polymers are becoming potential candidate materials for implantable drug delivery system requiring sustained action.

The major degradation process of biodegradable polymers is either by bulk hydrolysis or by enzymatic action. Zero order drug release rate kinetics is feasible with the use of biodegradable polymers, which are hydrophobic such as polyanhydrides and polyorthoesters. Changing the degradability of the carrier polymer can control the drug release rate. The advantage of using a degradable polymer is that the control dosage can be varied with a change in the polymer degradation rate and terminated with the elimination of the device (the carrier), once the required amount of drug is delivered.

11.5   Summary

Drug delivery is rapidly advancing beyond traditional practices such as oral ingestion and hypodermic injection. The two principal new modes of drug delivery are selective drug release to specific tissues or organs and controlled drug release to match the immediate needs of the patient for e.g., insulin release. A range of new materials, mostly polymers, some artificial and some natural in original are being developed for the new forms of drug release. These polymers typically serve as an encapsulation that allows the drug to slowly escape into the tissues by diffusion. The service characteristics of these encapsulation materials are still largely unknown despite their evident importance.

References

You Han Bae and Sung Wan Kim, Drug delivery, In Frontiers in tissue engineering, editors., 1998, Pergamon Press, Elsevier Science, p 261.

Bioartificial organs II Technology, Medicine and Materials, Ed. David Hunkeler, Ales Prokop, Allan D. Cherrington, Ray V. Rajotte, and Michael Sefton, Annals of New York Academy of Sciences, 1999, Vol. 875, Parts 1-7, pp. 71-254.

Ian Sample, Bullets from a tiny plasma gun can unclog the blocked veins that threaten eyesight, New Scientist, Online News, 25 April 2001.

Michael V. Sefton et al., Immunoisolation, in Frontiers in tissue engineering, editors. Charles W. Patrick Jr., A.G.Mikos & L.V.McIntire., 1998, Pergramon Press, Elsevier Science, p 248.

C.T. Vogelson, Advances in drug delivery systems, ACS Publications, Focus: Nanotechnology, April 2001, Vol. 4, pp. 49-50, 52.

http://pubs.acs.org/subscribe/journals/mdd/v04/i04/html/MDD04Feature Vogelson.html

http://www.nih.gov/od/ors/dbeps/ddkr/index.htm

http://www.medscape.com

Chapter 12

Physiological Reaction to Medical Instrumentation and Disposal of Used Biomaterials

12.1 Introduction

Medical Instrumentation is known interact with the human subject to produce harmful side effects. An early example of a harm interaction is Rontgen's experience with X-rays, after he had irradiated his hand to collect an image of the bones within the hand; he developed sores on his hands. These were later known to have resulted from excessive X-ray exposure. Any form of instrumentation, which involves insertion of a device within the human body, will carry a risk of transmitted infection. A common example is the thermometer, which is now sheathed in a disposable plastic cover. In order to ensure that the benefits of medical instrumentation outweigh any dangers, it is necessary to be able to manage the risks of harmful interaction between the patient and a medical instrument.

Medical treatment, like almost any other human enterprise, generates waste. This waste is growing in quantity and diversity and is creating a disposal problem. It has been estimated that the length of kidney dialysis tubing disposed annually totals 150 million km [Vienken, 2000]. This distance is approximately the same as the distance between the sun and the earth, which is shown schematically in Figure 12.1.

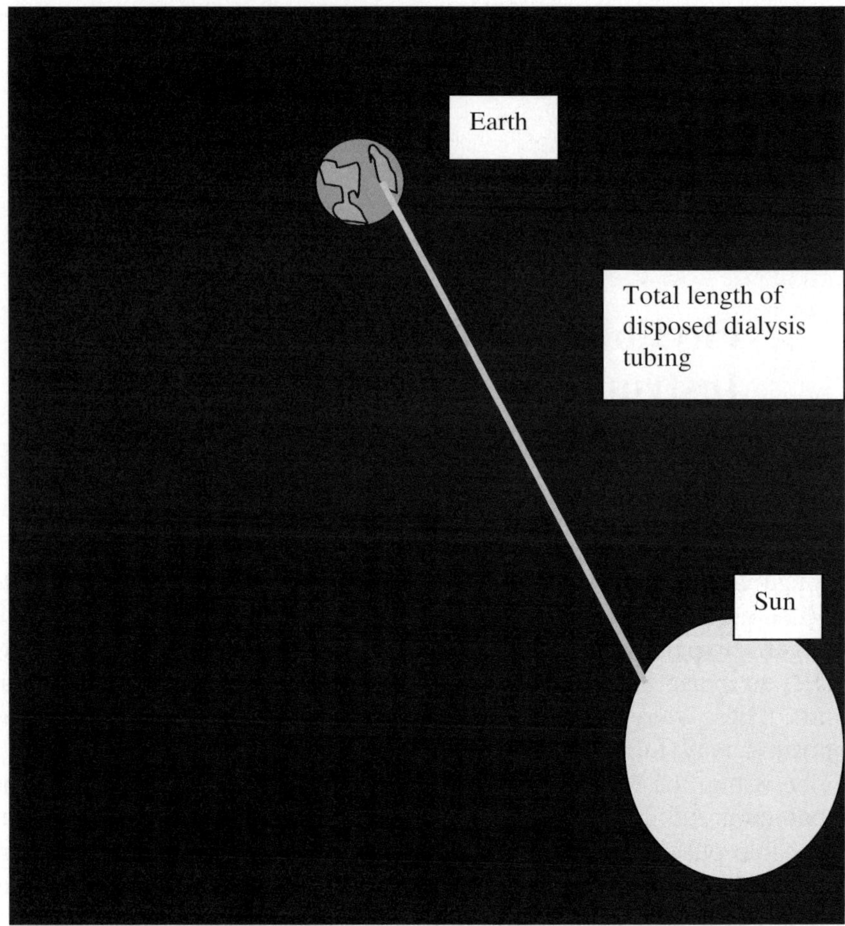

Fig 12.1. An astronomical comparison of an estimate of the length of kidney dialysis tubing used and disposed of annually.

12.2 Endoscopes

Endoscopes are a rapidly growing in scope and type. The conventional endoscope, which involves a camera attached to a tube, is being supplemented by autonomous endoscopes. These endoscopes, which are constructed as capsules with enclosed electronic sensors, offer a much wider range of data about the patient. The small size of these autonomous endoscopes, allows the patient to be spared the pain caused by passage of a tube through the human gut or bladder. The material used for the capsule should be non-toxic, non-allergenic and corrosion-resistant. Corrosion-resistance will be critical for endoscopy of the stomach where very high acidities prevail. The possibility of an autonomous endoscope becoming trapped in the patient should also be considered. To provide for this eventuality, the capsule material should be selected for very high levels of non-toxicity, non-allergenicity and corrosion resistance. The size and shape of the endoscope should also be controlled, sharp edges and projecting tips could cause damage to internal tissues.

Nitinol a super-elastic material also finds use in endoscopes especially when the complications associated with endoscopic operations increase. The super elastic nature of nitinol permits insertion of a complex instrument through a relatively narrow and straight trocar. However, when biocompatibility is considered nitinol itself is highly biocompatible and considered to be stable and corrosion resistant. But on the other hand oxidation of nitinol produces Titanium Dioxide and microscopic 'islands' of pure nickel in the remaining metal, which are considered to be toxic. Hence sufficient care should be exercised to avoid circumstances that might lead to oxidation of nitinol in the endoscopic tooling [Duerig et al., 1996].

Other form of problems associated with endoscopic procedures are splenic trauma, vasovagal reactions and endocarditis. Sepsis and other infections following colonoscopy (a form of endoscopy) are rare.

12.3   Biosensors

Biosensors are gaining prominence over the past two decades due to the developments in the field of bioengineering and drug delivery systems. The primary functions of a biosensor are to sense and signal to the mimetic organs for either triggering a release of a hormone or a drug or provide necessary data for monitoring the functionality of an organ or an implant. They consist of sensing elements, which consist of one of opto-electronic, bio-infrared or enzyme-based devices. They can be typically cell-based biosensors on a silicon substrate or involve other modes of sensing. A typical example of natural bio sensing is the secretion of insulin depending on the glucose levels in humans. If the designated cell or drug is not released to suit the physiological responses, it defeats the purpose of the cell / drug delivery. In order to fulfill the functional requirements of a sensor, it has to meet certain requirements. It should be biocompatible, should not be identified by the host tissue as a foreign body to avoid any rejections and not react with the physiological medium to change the properties of the device material other than those intended [Hunkeler et al., 2001].

12.4   Ultra-sound and Magnetic Resonance Imaging

Ultrasound and Magnetic Resonance imaging (MRI) are used for the imaging of soft tissues with significant water content. Both these imaging techniques are non-invasive and without major hazards. However, MRI is found to involve more risks than Ultrasound imaging. Magnetic resonance imaging has been used extensively in the field for medicine for diagnostics in Cardio vascular, orthopedic, neurology, vascular besides being used for spectroscopy and interventional purposes. Certain safety requirements has to be taken in to consideration while using MRI for specific diagnostic purposes in patients such as strength of the magnetic field, rate change of the magnetic field and absorption rate of radio frequency by the patients body. Besides these functional issues MRI image quality is affected by the other factors such as interference from pace makers in the vicinity of the MRI units, presence of extraneous objects like surgical clips or implants. Any implants, which are likely to become affected by the magnetic field, can cause serious consequences for patients. A typical example of such problems is the case of a slight movement of an inter-cranial aneurysm clip while being exposed to static magnetic field. Similar cases have also been reported on the insulin pump being non-functional upon exposure to Pulsed Radio Frequencies. Some of the devices, which are termed Passive devices in MRI terminology, are the aneurysm clips, shunts, oxygen bottles, Scalpels and IV poles. These typically fulfil their function without the supply of power. These are only examples of typical hazards caused by MRI in patients with implants or other medical devices. A wealth of information on the MRI related safety measures with respect to implants, medical devices (such as pacemakers) is provided by the US FDA web site http://www.fda.gov/cdrh/ode/primerf6.html .

Ultrasound is another typical device, which is widely used for diagnostics similar to MRI. However, the effect of materials on ultrasound and the vice versa are less serious compared to MRI. The most important requirement of an ultrasound device with respect to its service is that the sensors or transducers used should be biocompatible and should not cause any allergies to the patient.

12.5 Radiology

Radiology is widely used in medicine for imaging of human tissues to facilitate diagnosis. The most common form of radiology is X-ray imaging where a Rontgen X-ray source is used to produce a beam of X-rays that passes through the human body. An image of tissue is obtained from the variation in X-ray adsorption between different tissues. Bones, which contain calcium, show the highest adsorption levels and are the most clearly imaged tissues. The X-ray system is non-invasive, rapidly generates images and is mechanically reliable. There is no strict need for physical contact between the patient and X-ray imaging system, so cross-infection risks between patients can be controlled. However, in many X-ray imaging systems, patients are expected to rest themselves against an imaging plate. For these systems, if there were a cross-infection risk, it would be possible to cover the imaging plate with a disposable plastic membrane, or disinfect the imaging plate after each patient. The critical limitation of X-ray imaging is the harmful effect of ionizing radiation on human cells. X-ray exposure has to be carefully limited and this restricts the number of images that can be collected from a patient over any given period of time. There are many historical examples of radiographers who died from X-ray induced cancers because they did not wear adequate protective clothing and did not control their X-ray exposure [University of Iowa].

In addition to the radiological induced damages such as cell damage for low doses to very high doses causing permanent injury as elaborated above, implants also play a vital role in deciding the quality of the image obtained. Metallic implants may affect the quality of X-ray image by being radio-opaque (i.e. opaque to X-rays) while polymeric implants are often radio-transparent. Exposure of polymeric implants such as those used for tissue scaffolding to ionizing radiation may result in the deterioration of their material properties. In patients who have received either a transplanted organ or tissue scaffold organ regeneration, a low or medium dose of ionizing radiation would cause substantial damage to these organs.

Acrylic cements often lack sufficient radio-opacity for surgeons to be able to observe the characteristics of the cement that bonds an orthopaedic prosthesis to the surrounding bone. A method of increasing radio-opacity to acrylic cement is to mix in barium sulphate, however this may adversely affect the mechanical strength of the cement. A new additive to enhance radio-opacity is 4-iodophenol methacrylate (IPMA). A 15 weight % blend of IPMA in acrylic cement was found to provide the same radio-opacity as a 10 weight % blend of barium sulphate but with superior values of compressive, tensile strengths and elastic modulus [Artola et al., 2003]. Tissue reactions to the IPMA blend are also reported as favourable [Artola et al., 2003].

12.6   Waste disposal of used biomaterials

Waste disposal of used biomaterials is classified as medical waste if the biomaterials are used in the treatment of humans or of animals. If the biomaterial is only used in experiments not involving animal or human subjects, then it is not medical waste. The World Health Organization [Larkin, 2001], has stated the problem of safe disposal of health-care waste has the potential to reduce the overall benefits from health-care. To facilitate efficient disposal of health-care waste, the WHO has set up a working committee to provide guidance and information on medical waste. The disposal of medical waste is subject to various laws to prevent careless disposal. A range of government agencies, which regulate the various aspects of disposal, controls waste disposal procedures. For example, in the United States, the Environmental Protection Agency regulates the use of incinerators while the Department of Transportation regulates the transport of medical wastes.

The main requirement for safe disposal of medical wastes is the destruction of pathogenic organisms before release into the wider environment. Medical waste is sterilized by incineration or autoclaving before it is sent to the rubbish tip. There are other hazards associated with medical waste such as cuts from used hypodermic needles, lancets, scalpels and broken glass petri dishes. These items are usually disposed of in a bin that is separate from the bins used for general wastes. The disposal of medical wastes is usually entrusted to trained personnel in a hospital environment. However many medical materials, e.g. hypodermic needles for insulin injection have to be disposed off by the patients themselves. In this case, specially designed technology is needed to ensure the safe disposal of large quantities of insulin hypodermic needles. A device using electrical current to melt and disintegrate the needles has been recently devised and approved by the Food and Drug Administration of the United States of America [CDRH, 2002].

Some biomaterials can be recycled for profit; many orthopaedic prostheses are made of titanium alloys or other expensive metals. Used prostheses obtained from surgical revision can be returned to the metal foundry after sterilization. Adequate sterilization and cleaning is essential for safe re-use of prostheses and surgical tools. Complete sterilization of a surface is not easily achieved. As mentioned in Chapter 4, gamma-ray sterilization is practiced to sterilize orthopaedic implants but this process requires specialized equipment and is hazardous to personnel. Simpler forms of sterilization involve disinfectants. The most reliable disinfectant is sodium hypochlorite while other disinfectants and detergents are only partially effective [Meritt et al., 2000]. The latter disinfectants and detergents are unable to destroy bacteria that form strong biofilms such as Candida albicans. Any surface, which has been allowed to become dry, is the most difficult to disinfect.

Tonsillectomy (surgical removal of tonsils) is now performed using disposable surgical instruments to prevent cross-infection between patients, despite the self-evident increase in medical waste from used surgical tools. This practice has been adopted because of the risk of infection by the abnormal (mis-folded) prion proteins that cause the variant Creutzfeldt-Jakob disease [The Lancet, 2001]. It has been estimated that a dose of only 10,000 mis-folded prion proteins, weighing approximately 1 fg (1.0 E-15 g) are sufficient to infect a human patient [Bolton, 2001]. Mis-folded prions have been found not only in the nervous system but also in the lymph nodes and tonsils. This means that if even a truly minute speck of extracted tissue remains on a surgical instrument, there is a hazard for the next patient.

12.6.1 *Waste disposal problems during the manufacture of biomedical materials*

The manufacture of biomedical materials may generate almost as many problems of toxic waste as the final disposal itself. Polyvinyl chloride (PVC) is used in many medical products such as intravenous bags, tubing and blood bags. The manufacture of PVC involves toxic chemicals such as 1,2 - dichloroethane and releases dioxin, which is a very hazardous material [Healing the harm]. Incineration, which is a widely used practice for medical waste, becomes hazardous when PVC is collected. Incineration of PVC generates dioxins and hydrochloric acid, which is destructive of incineration equipment.

12.6.2 *Disposal of dental amalgams*

As discussed in Chapter 6, dental amalgam is classified as a hazardous material because of its mercury content. This poses problems in its routine disposal from dental clinics. It has been estimated that approximately 75 tons of dental amalgam are extracted annually from patients in the USA [Osborne, 1992]. With many more tons of dental amalgam residing in the mouths of patients. Dental clinics have been isolated as a significant source of mercury release into the environment [Fan et al., 1997]. The current method of preventing uncontrolled amalgam release is to insert filters into the suction systems and basins of the dental clinic.   Placement of dental amalgam in a patient's teeth involves the release of many particles of amalgam. These particles may either be collected by the suction lines that drain the patients mouth or from the basin when the patient is instructed to spit out after treatment. In either location, it is important than an effective filter is present. Specialized companies offer a service of collecting the filters for controlled disposal. However, it may also be noted that a significant amount of dental amalgam is lost inadvertently during eating and presumably finds its way into the public sewage system.

12.6.3 *Disposal of kidney dialysis systems*

Kidney dialysis waste represents a large and rapidly growing source of medical waste. The prime source of waste is the dialysis tubing, which is disposed in very large volumes. Although the dialysis tubing is not especially hazardous, the scale of disposal is beginning to present difficulties. A major difficulty is that the dialysis tubing, especially from peritoneal dialysis may contain infectious viruses. This means that the tubing has to be disinfected before disposal [PDServe].

A widely practiced means of reducing the costs of dialysis tubing is to the re-use of tubing that is intended as single-use by its manufacturer [Health Devices]. Frequent re-use of dialysis tubing may lead to its cracking during service; cracked tubing would then cause blood loss by the patient. In some cases, immediate blood transfusion was required to compensate for this blood loss. The cause of the cracking is attributed to degradation of the tubing material during washing with disinfectants and to the practice of tapping the dialysis pack with a hard object to dislodge bubbles from inside the tubing. Trapped bubbles would be deadly to a patient if they remained in the dialyzer. If the tubing material is made of polycarbonate, aromatic compounds in some types of disinfectant can react with the polycarbonate to cause embrittlement. Disinfectants based on strong oxidizers such as hypochlorite would also cause eventual degradation of the polycarbonate.

12.7   Re-use of biomaterials

The high cost of many implanted medical devices, e.g. US$10,000 for a pacemaker, has provoked many parties to consider re-use of expensive medical devices after the patient no longer needs them. One proposal was to remove the device from the body of a dead patient and reuse it, assuming that the device (e.g. a pacemaker) was still functional. The high cost of medical technology has created a strong practical need for re-use even where the original purpose was only for single use such as balloon catheters for coronary angioplasty [Plante et al.].

Some medical devices can be recycled after the original user has outlived their usefulness. Orthodontic metal braces are an example of recycling, however this practice has been found to be associated with several health incidents [Lewis, 2000]. In the United States of America, the Food and Drug Administration (FDA) now requires healthcare facilities to record the receipt, distribution and final disposal of many medical devices [Murphy, 2002]. Devices listed by the FDA include the cardiovascular permanent implantable pacemaker electrode and the implantable pacemaker pulse generator.

Some major considerations are (i) sterilization of the used medical device without destroying its continued functioning, (ii) the materials stability in the medical device may only be sufficient for use by a single patient, (iii) liability of manufacturer or recycler if there is a subsequent health problem for the new user. There appears to have been limited consideration of sterilization by the parties involved in recycling. For most electronic devices, extreme heat or pressurized steam sterilization would be destructive to the device. Irradiation by gamma rays would also almost certainly degrade either the casing of the electronic device or else the circuits within. These restrictions leave only room temperature sterilization with bactericidal gases such as ethylene oxide. The question of leakage of entrapped toxic gases from recesses inside the electronic device would remain to be addressed.

The monolithic components used to form orthopaedic implants such as the hip prosthesis may appear to be attractive to recycle. Orthopaedic implants are expensive and their monolithic structure would facilitate sterilization when compared to the hollow recessed structure of a probe or electronic device. The recycling of hip prostheses would involve problems such as: (i) the very high level of sterility required for orthopaedic implants, (ii) scratching or other mechanical damage to the implant during recycling would render it unsuitable for further use, (iii) the stem of the implant is fitted individually to the femur of each patient, recycling would lose the required fit.

To conclude, the altruistic purpose of allowing a less fortunate patient to enjoy the benefits of a recycled implant at lower cost than a new implant is rendered invalid by the dangers inherent. Most re-used single devices are surgical instruments such as a surgical saw blade, umbilical scissors and balloon angioplasty catheter [Lewis].

The issue of whether to re-use or dispose used medical devices remains an issue of widespread concern [Collignon et al., 1996]. Much medical equipment and devices used in surgical procedures are designed as Single Use Devices (SUDs). SUDs have been re-used in various hospitals where it is assumed that the quality of sterilization is adequate to ensure the safety of patients. Sterilization of SUDs is impeded by the design of the devices, which often contain numerous recesses, crevices and holes [Collignon et al., 1996]. Such crevices and recesses impede mechanical cleaning of deposits of e.g., blood.   Hardened deposits are not easily penetrated by ethylene oxide, thereby allowing a sheltered niche to remain for micro-organisms [Collignon et al., 1996]. Ethylene oxide is a toxic gas that is widely used to sterilize medical devices.

Another aspect of recycling that deserves mention is the role of the sterilization process. Ethylene oxide is widely used to sterilize devices such as catheters. Where repeated recycling is practiced, there is a concern that ethylene oxide would accumulate in the sterilized devices and exceed the safe limits for ethylene oxide [Lucas et al., 2003]. Polymers are known to absorb ethylene oxide, where high levels of absorption are associated with increased crystallinity in the polymer. Polymers were found to vary widely in their absorption of ethylene oxide, with common polymers such as Nylon 66 showing the highest levels of ethylene oxide uptake [Lucas et al., 2003]. A mitigating factor to the toxicity of ethylene oxide was found to be a lower level of 'bioavailability' compared to the chemical concentration in the polymer. Bioavailability is defined as the amount of substance made available to living human cells.

12.8 Summary

The problem of disposing of used medical devices is growing in complexity and size as the number of users rapidly increases. Some medical problems such as those made of PVC pose environmental risks, while others such as hypodermic needles become dangerous after use. Specialized technology is being devised to safely dispose of popular items. Medical instrumention and endoscopes also impose risks, although small, such as effects on previously installed implants.

References

David C Bolton, Prions and proteins: distinguishing between conformations, The Lancet, Vol. 358, No. 9277, 21 July 2001
http://www.thelancet.com/journal/vol358/iss92.../llan.358.9277.editorial and_review.16958

CDRH Consumer Information, New Device Approval – Disintegrator™ Insulin Needle Destruction Unit P010040, 22 March 2002, http://www.fda.gov/cdrh/mda/docs/p010040.html

T.W. Duerig, A.R. Pelton and D. Stockel, 1996, The use of Superelasticity in Medicine, METALL Sonderdruck aus Heft 9/96, pp. 569-574, Metall Verlag –Huthig GmbH, Heidelberg, Germany.

P.L. Fan, D. Arenholt-Bindstv, G. Schmalz, S. Halbach and H. Berendsen, Environmental issues in dentistry - mercury, FDI World Dental Federation International Dental Journal, 1997, Vol. 47, No. 2, pp. 105-109.

Peter J. Collignon, Elaine Graham and Dianne E. Dreimanis, 1996, Reuse in sterile sites of single-use devices: How common is this in Australia? The Medical Journal of Australia, Vol. 164, pp. 533-536.

Header Cracks Related to Reprocessing of Single-Use Hemodialysis Dialyzers, Health Devices, Aug-Sep 1995, Vol. 24, No. 8-9, pp. 359-361.

Healing the Harm: Eliminating the pollution from health care practices, "Section Six: Creating a materials policy to minimize pollution". http://www.sustain.org/hcwh/hcwhmanual/hthmedpvc.html

David Hunkeler, Alan Cherrington, Alex Prokop & Ray Rajotte et al.editors, 2001, Bioartificial organs III, Tissue Sourcing, Immunoisolation and clinical trials, Annals of New York Academy of Sciences, Vol. 944, 2001, pp 18-34, 83-95.

Marilyn Larkin, *Click of the week*, Managing health-care waste, The Lancet, Vol. 357, No. 9272, 16 June 2001. http://www.thelancet.com/journal/vol357/iss9272/full/llan.357.9272.diss ecting_room.16571.3

C. Lewis, Reusing Medical Devices: Ensuring Safety The Second Time Around, FDA Consumer Magazine, September – October 2000, http://www.fad.gov/fdac/features/2000/500_resue.html

A.D. Lucas, K. Merritt, V.M. Hitchins, T.O. Woods, S.G. McNamee, D.B. Lyle and S.A. Brown, Residual ethylene oxide in medical devices and device material, Journal of Biomedical Materials Research, Part B: Applied Biomaterials, 2003, Vol. 66B, No. 2, pp. 548-552.

K. Merritt, V.M. Hitchins and S.A. Brown, Safety and cleaning of medical materials and devices, Journal of Biomedical Materials Research, 2000, Vol. 53, No. 2, pp. 131-136.

S. Murphy, ECRI Reissues FDA's List of Tracked Medical Devices, ECRI Press, 7th March 2002,
http://www.ecri.org/documents/030702.asp

J.W. Osborne, Dental Amalgam and Mercury Vapor Release, Advances in Dental Research, 1992, September, Vol. 6, pp. 135-138.

PD Serves, Issues in Peritoneal Dialysis Infection Control,
http://www.pdserve.com/pdserve/pdserve.nsf/Content/Vol.+2%C+No.1

S. Plante, B.H. Strauss, G. Goulet, R.K. Watson and R.J. Chisholm, Reause of balloon catheters for coronary angioplasty: A potential cost saving strategy? Journal of the American College of Cardiology, 1994, Vol. 24, pp. 1475-1481.

Prions revealed, Talking points, The Lancet, Vol. 358, No. 9277, 21 July 2001
http://www.thelancet.com/journal/vol358/iss9277/full/llan.358.9277.talk king_points.16983.5

University of Iowa Health care, Medical Museum, The trail of invisible light: A century of medical imaging, X-ray martyrs.
http://www.uihealthcare.com/depts/medmuseum/trailoflight/03xraymarty rs.html

Jorg Vienken, Polymers in Nephrology: Needs, properties and performance, Proc. 10th International Conference on Biomedical Engineering, 6-9th December 2000, Singapore, edit. J.C.H. Goh, publ. National University of Singapore,

World Health Organization, Health-Care Waste Working Group. http://www.healthcarewaste.org/htmlpages/welcomeEntry.html

P.L. Fan, D. Arenholt-Bindstv, G. Schmalz, S. Halbach and H. Berendsen, Environmental issues in dentistry - mercury, FDI World Dental Federation International Dental Journal, 1997, Vol. 47, No. 2, pp. 105-109.

J.W. Osborne, Dental Amalgam and Mercury Vapor Release, Advances in Dental Research, 1992, September, Vol. 6, pp. 135-138.

Artola, I. Goni, P. Ginebra, J.M. Manero and M. Gurruchaga, A radiopaque polymeric matrix for acrylic bone cements, Journal of Biomedical Materials Research, Part B, Applied Biomaterials, 2003, Vol. 64B, No. 1, pp. 44-55.

Government and Technical Society Standards for Biomedical Materials

Since the health of patients and the liability of medical personnel are involved, it is apparent that legally enforceable standards are a prerequisite for the safe use of implants.   The need for systematic testing and evaluation of the hazards of biomaterials was given formal recognition by Autian [Autian] in 1961. Autian proposed a series of *in vivo* tests on model animals, which would be used to estimate the level of hazard to humans. Standardized tests for manufacturers are based on a scheme arising from Autian's work where a range of representative tissues are chosen for testing. An implant manufacturer has to then select the appropriate 'matrix', e.g., human tissue or external material, the tissue type that contacts the implant and the duration of implantation. The duration of implantation and the tissue type are therefore the primary parameters for hazards testing. Instead of seeking to quantify hazards levels, a confirmation of satisfactory performance termed 'biocompatibility' is the accepted parameter. Biocompatibility means that a biomedical material or a biomedical device does not pose a significant risk to patients.

Safety is an elusive quantity to define since it involves unknown hazards, but for the purpose of certifying biomedical devices the following definition of safety is applied. The safety of device is considered to the sum of its chemical, microbiological and physical safety [Kuijpers and Dorpema]. The basic risks are toxicity, carcinogenic risk, genotoxicity, sensitisation (allergic response) and thrombosis (for implants contacting blood). Infection by bacterially contaminated implants is not usually tested because of the severe sterilisation processes that implants are subjected to. However, the hazards associated with sterilization, e.g., residual ethylene (a sterilizing agent) are the subject of tests.

The management of biomaterials has been assumed by governmental authorities such as the Food and Drug Administration (FDA) in the USA with standardised test protocols specified by the International Standards Organization (ISO) and the American Society for the Testing of Materials (ASTM). Relevant standards are the F748 standard issued by the F04 ASTM committee on medical and surgical devices and materials, the ISO 10993 entitled 'Biological evaluation of medical devices' and EN 30993 of the European Committee for Standardisation (CEN). EN 30993 closely corresponds to ISO 10993 while there is only partial agreement between these and the ASTM standards. It is important to note that these standards primarily relate to biomedical devices as opposed to biomedical materials. It is conceivable that a material, which is harmless when implanted alone, may become toxic in combination with other biomedical materials. A possible scenario is a galvanic cell formed between contacting dissimilar metals that leads to the release of carcinogenic metal ions from an otherwise inert metal.

The application of standards to biomedical materials and devices is a complex process involving legal as well as technical issues. A review of this subject is provided by Marlowe [Marlowe] and Kujpers and Dorpema [Kujpers and Dorpema]. A major problem for implant manufacturers is conflicting requirements of different national regulatory agencies. Within Europe, this problem has largely been overcome by the adoption of the CEN directives.

The ISO 10993 is divided into 12 parts, which specify all relevant aspects of testing for biocompatibility [Marlowe]. The 12 parts are listed below:

Part 1   Guidance on selection of tests
Part 2 Animal welfare requirements
Part 3 Tests for genotoxicity, carcinogenicity and reproductive toxicity
Part 4 Selection of tests for interaction with blood
Part 5 Tests for cytotoxicity, in vitro methods
Part 6 Tests for local effects after implantation
Part 7 Ethylene oxide sterilisation residues

Part 8 Clinical investigation (not part of EN 30993)
Part 9 Degradation of materials related to biological testing
Part 10 Tests for irritation and sensitisation
Part 11 Tests for systemic toxicity
Part 12 Sample preparation and reference materials

While very detailed, it should be noted that ISO 10993 does not specifically cover recognized problems such as the inflammation induced by wear debris [Gott]. All standards will need to be continuously extended and revised as new devices enter the biomedical market. For example, resorbable 'scaffolds' present new risks and requirements for testing.

There are also other pertinent ISO standards with extra provisions for dental materials.   Important ISO standards include: ISO 5832-2: 1993 Implants for Surgery – Metallic Materials – Part 2: Unalloyed titanium, ISO 5832-3: 1996 Implants for Surgery – Metallic Materials – Part 3: Wrought Titanium 6 – Aluminium 4 – Vanadium alloy, ISO 7405: 1997 Dentistry – Pre-clinical Evaluation of Biocompatibility of Medical Devices used in Dentistry – Test Methods for Dental Materials. As can be seen, dental materials and prostheses have their own specialized testing requirements, which are not applicable to other implants. Further information about dental materials, especially endosseous dental implants is provided by the web page of the FDA, Center for Devices and Radiological Health.

References

J. Autian, Plastics: uses and problems in pharmacy and medicine, American Journal of Hospital Pharmacy, 1961, Vol. 18, pp. 329-249.

Don Marlowe, Biocompatibility standards: An international overview, Part 1: United States, in **Biocompatibility Assessment of Medical Devices and Materials,** editor Julian H. Braybrook, John Wiley and Sons, Chichester, United Kingdom, 1997, pp. 1-8.

Marja Kujpers and Jan-Willem Dorpema, Biocompatibility Standards: An international overview, Part 2: Europe, in **Biocompatibility Assessment of Medical Devices and Materials**, editor Julian H. Braybrook, John Wiley and Sons, Chichester, United Kingdom, 1997, pp. 9-19.

David Gott, Biodegradation and toxicokinetic studies, Biocompatibility Assessment of Medical Devices and Materials, editor Julian H. Braybrook, John Wiley and Sons, Chichester, United Kingdom, 1997, pp. 43-63.

U.S. Department of Health and Human Services, Food and Drug Administration, Center for Devices and Radiological Health, Dental Device Branch, Division of Dental, Infection Control and General Hospital Devices, 14th May 2002,
http://www.fda.gov/cdrh/ode/guidance/1389.html

APPENDIX 2

Experimental Apparatus to Measure the Service Characteristics of Implants

There is a wide variety of specialized apparatus to measure the service characteristics of biomaterials. Some of the most elaborate apparatus relate to predicting the wear characteristics of biomaterials. Experimental measurements of the long-term wear characteristics of orthopaedic prostheses such as the hip implant represent perhaps the greatest experimental challenge. Accelerated testing is required to simulate 20 years of service in as short a period as 6 months. This is a 40-fold acceleration over the natural rate of service and is possibly close to the limit where over-heating would compromise the quality of wear simulation. Polymer wear is very strongly influenced by frictionally induced temperature elevation. Finger implants are tested to measure the fatigue life before breakage of the implant where elastic flexure permits rotation or wear when the implant is articulated. The wear of heart valves is tested for fracture and wear in an apparatus that simulates the flow of blood through the heart with repeated opening and closing of the valve. The figures below show some representative examples of apparatus. There is a wide range of apparatus so some important devices have been omitted. An important example of this is the multi-channel hip implant tester, which allows e.g., 12, hip specimens to be tested together for greater speed of data collection.

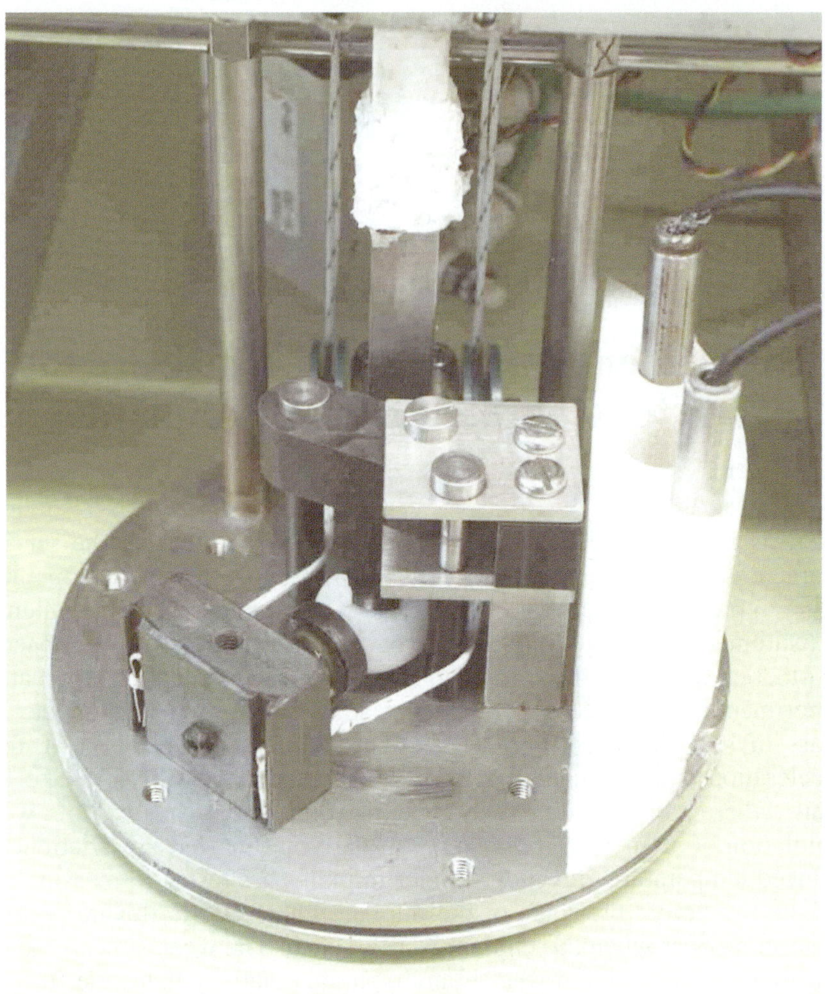

Fig A2.1. Detail view of an apparatus to test finger implants.
Picture provided by courtesy of Dr Tom Joyce, Centre for Biomedical Engineering, University of Durham, Great Britain.

The friction and wear of the sliding joint of a finger implant is measured using this Ball-on-cup apparatus. Polymers such as Ultra High Molecular Weight Polyethylene are subjected to reciprocating rotation against a smooth, hard metal counter face. The white coloured cords connect the cup to a drive system. This apparatus provides basic information allowing estimates of the wear of the rotating joint in a finger implant.

The overall view of the apparatus is shown below, where the drive system can be clearly seen.

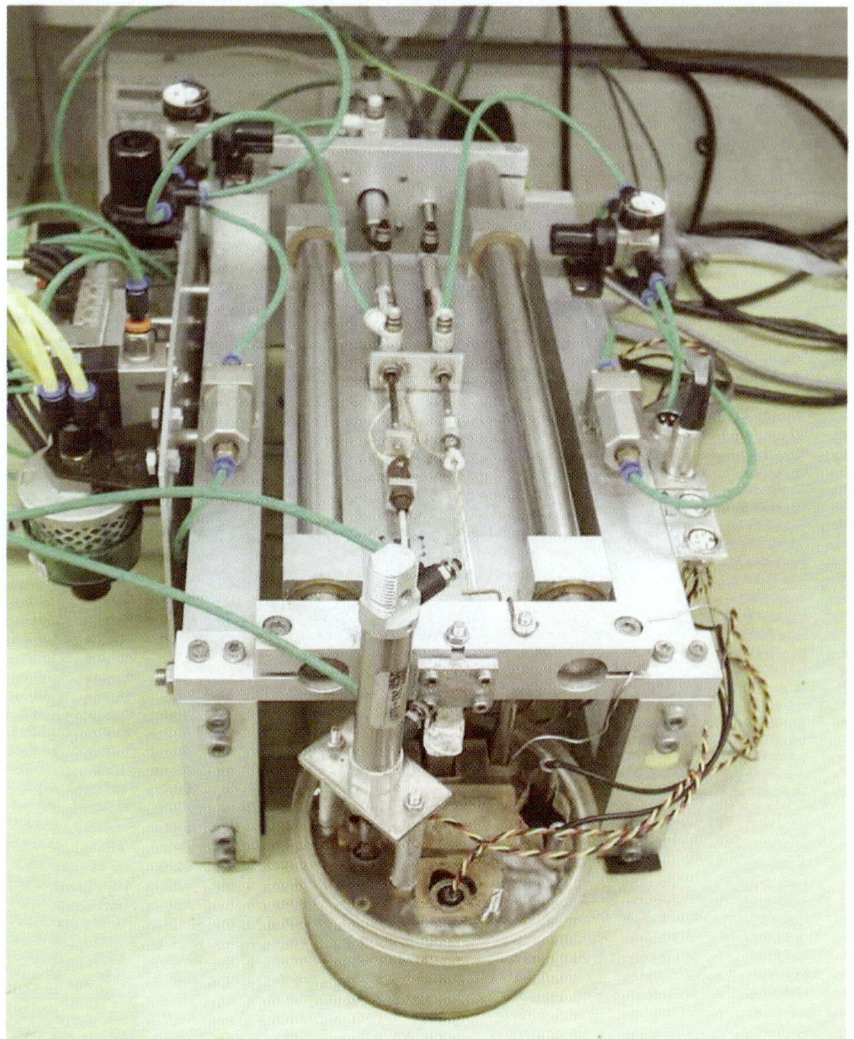

Fig A2.2.   General view of finger implant apparatus.Picture provided by courtesy of Dr Tom Joyce, University of Durham, Centre for Biomedical Engineering, Great Britain.

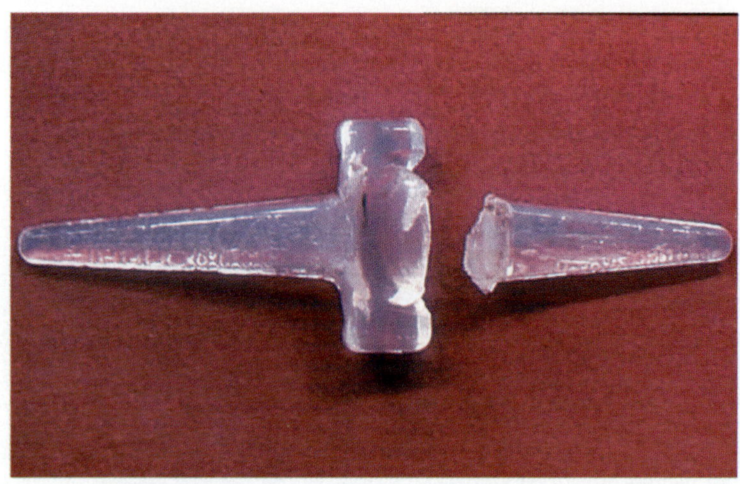

Fig A2.3.   Swanson type implant where rotation is generated by elastic bending. Fracture after repeated flexure during a test. Picture provided by courtesy of Dr Tom Joyce, Centre for Biomedical Engineering, University of Durham, Great Britain.

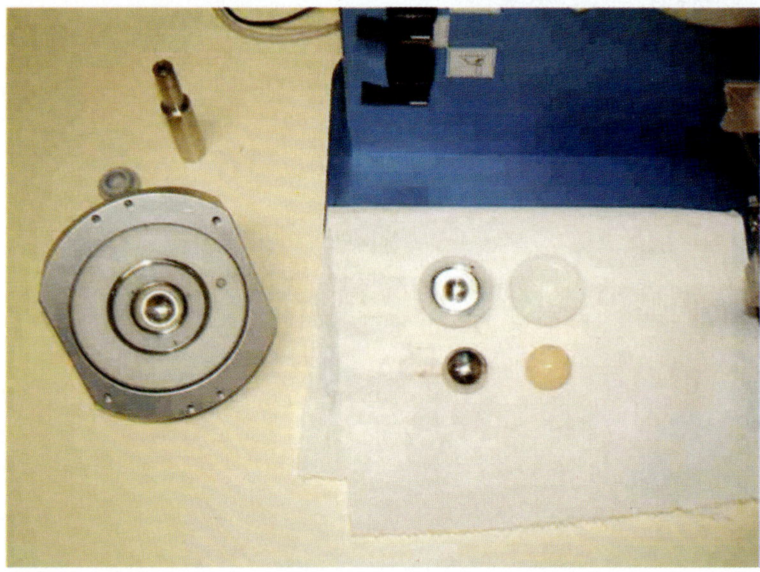

Fig A2.4.   Hip ball and cup specimens for an implant wear test. Picture provided by courtesy of Prof. Dr.Dipl.Ing. Kurt P. Judmann and Dipl.Ing. Georg Reinisch of Vienna University of Technology and the BMF Biomechanische Forschungs-Gesellschaft m.b.H, Vienna, Austria.

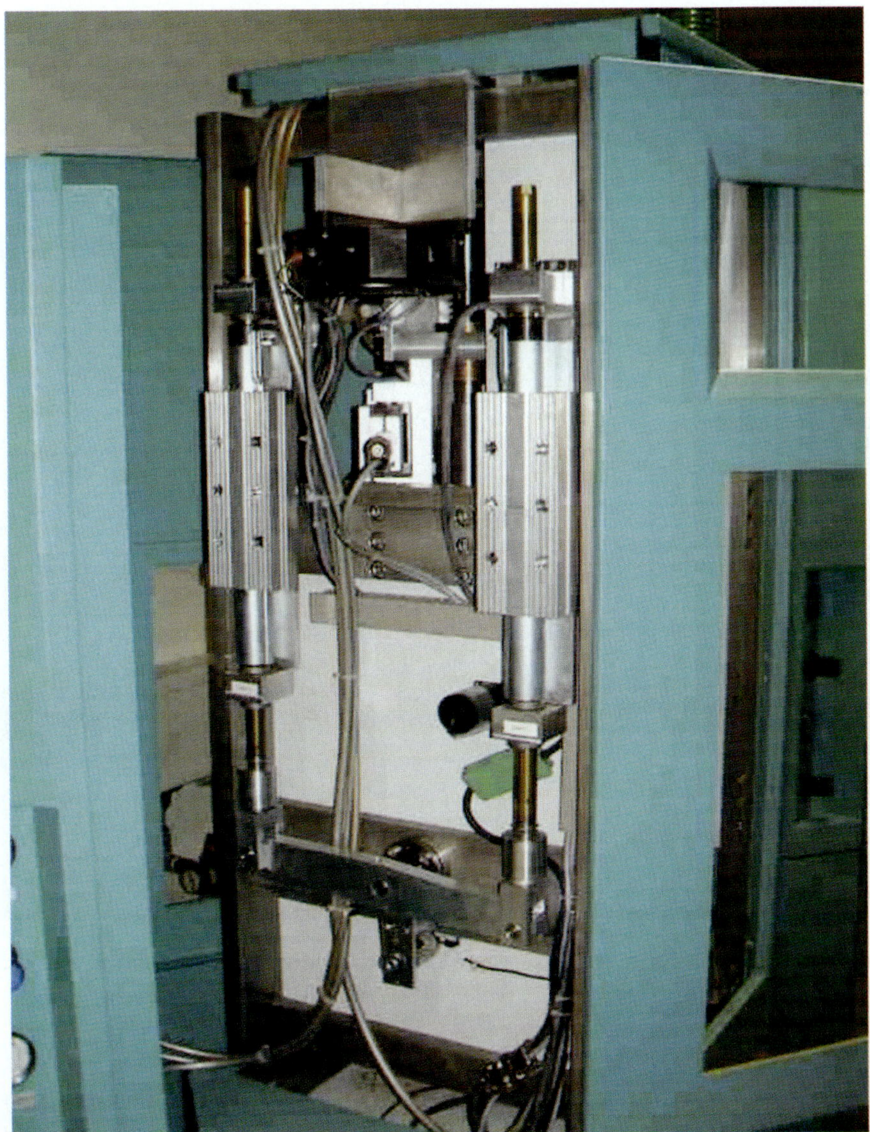

Fig A2.5.   General view of the hip implant tester. Picture provided by courtesy of Prof. Dr.Dipl.Ing. Kurt P. Judmann and Dipl.Ing. Georg Reinisch of Vienna University of Technology and the BMF Biomechanische Forschungs-Gesellschaft m.b.H, Vienna, Austria.

This apparatus delivers reciprocating motion and variable loading that closely simulates the loads and forces encountered during normal walking. The high quality of construction and instrumentation is necessary to ensure constant test conditions during weeks of continuous testing.

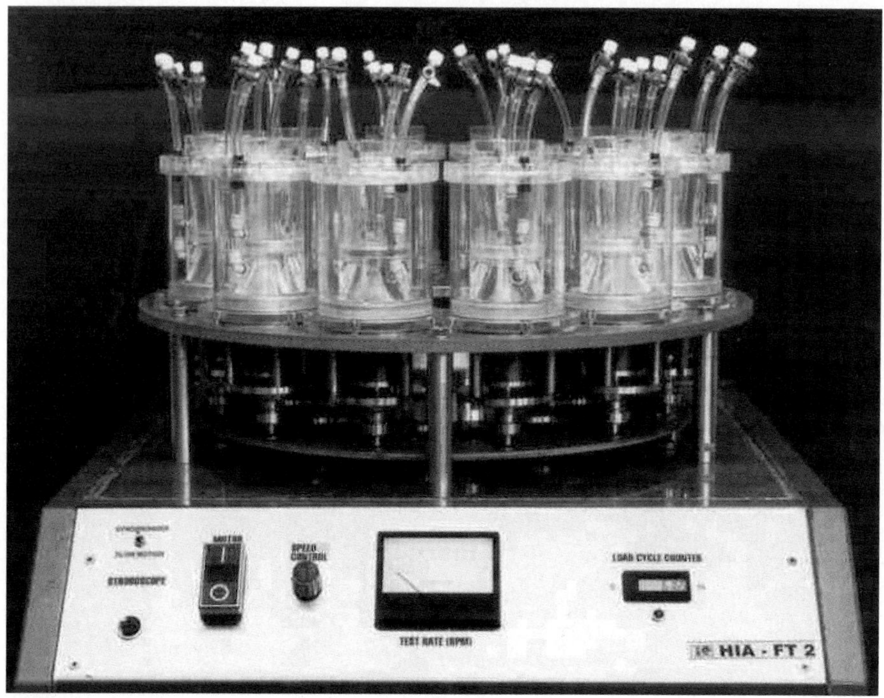

Fig A2.6.   Heart-valve tester. Picture provided by courtesy of Dr Wolfgang Kerkhoffs, Helmholtz-Institute of Biomedical Engineering, University of Technology, Aachen, Germany.

Heart valves are subjected to millions of closures and openings during service. A vital service characteristic, which must be tested experimentally, is resistance to fracture and wear. For basic testing (as opposed to testing in animal models and later, human volunteers), an oscillating flow of aqueous liquid is cycled through the valve until the required number of opening / closure cycles have been reached. The valves can then be removed to inspect for damage.

Index

V

VAD, 204
Vascular implants, 125
VCJD, 11
VEGF, 191
Vitallium^{TM}, 140

X

XRD, 202

Y

Yttrium, 153
Y-TZP, 73